Sciatica *Secrets*

Front Body Secret: Your back pain doesn't start in your back. Front body compression, psoas, iliacus, diaphragm, chest, creates the problem.

The Breathing Secret: Pranayama breathing releases your psoas-diaphragm-pelvic floor triad from inside. Ball work releases from outside. Also resets your nervous system.

The Diagonal Secret: Sciatica may come from cross-body patterns. Right shoulder compresses left hip. Left chest pulls right hip. Release the diagonals or hip work won't hold.

The Sleep Secret: Eight hours in wrong position re-shortens hip flexors every night. Discs are swollen and vulnerable first hour after waking. Adjust sleep position. Protect your morning.

The Opening Secret: Opening isn't stretching. Three to five minutes with breath integration teaches your nervous system the new length is safe and permanent.

The MRI Secret: Thirty to forty percent of pain-free people have disc abnormalities. Size of herniation doesn't predict pain. Structure doesn't equal symptoms.

The Triad Secret: Psoas, diaphragm, and pelvic floor work as one system. Can't release one without addressing all three.

The Forces Secret: You can be functional without structural healing. My structure didn't change. The forces acting on it did. That was enough.

The Symptom Secret: Sciatica describes nerve irritation. The cause is usually front-body compression. Fix the compression, quiet the nerve.

The 90 Day Secret: Ninety days is the minimum for fascia to remodel and neurological pathways to reinforce. After thirty days, habit forms. After sixty days, neural pathways

These secrets are revealed chapter by chapter throughout the book, then brought together in Chapter 14 with your complete 90-day protocol.

Sciatica *Secrets*

Back Pain Exposed Series, Book 1
backpainexposed.com

Medical Disclaimer:

This book is **for educational and informational purposes only** and is not intended as medical advice. The content is **based on the author's personal experience and professional practice** and should not replace consultation with qualified healthcare professionals. **Always consult your physician before beginning any new program,** especially if you have existing health conditions, or structural spinal issues. The author and publisher disclaim any liability for adverse effects arising from the use or application of the information contained in this book.

ISBN: 978-1-7390295-0-0
First Edition, 2025

Are You in Spasm Now?

CRITICAL: A true back spasm is a neurological emergency, not just a muscle cramp. The body's protective reflex system has locked down movement.

Emergency Actions for your First 24-48 Hours

Stop All Movement: No stretching, yoga, massage, or release work. Movement during acute spasm triggers more threat signals, intensifying the lock.

Find Positions of Comfort: Choose the least painful position:

- On your back: knees bent, pillow under knees
- On your side: pillow between knees
- Semi-reclined with knee support

Apply Continuous Heat.

Heat dilates blood vessels and signals the nervous system to shift from 'threat' mode to 'rest' mode. Use heating pad, hot water bottle, or warm bath continuously *(check skin every 20 minutes).*

Avoid ice in first 72 hours, cold increases muscle contraction.

Consider Muscle Relaxants.

Muscle relaxants work on the nervous system, not just the muscle, they dampen hyperexcitable spinal interneurons and reduce gamma motor neuron firing. Common options: methocarbamol *(Robaxin)*, cyclobenzaprine *(Flexeril)*, tizanidine *(Zanaflex)*. **Consult the healthcare provider in your area.**

Why they work: NSAIDs may reduce inflammation but won't break the spasm cycle. Muscle relaxants target the neurological lock at its source.

Breathe Gently: Soft belly breaths, inhale through nose, exhale through the mouth.

Hydrate with Electrolytes: Sip warm water throughout the day *(8+ glasses)*. Consider electrolytes, sodium, potassium, magnesium, which regulate muscle contraction and relaxation. Imbalances make muscles hyperexcitable.

Recovery Timeline: Acute spasms typically begin to ease within 3-7 days with proper rest. The first 72 hours are usually the hardest, then gradual release begins. **Full resolution may take 7-10 days.**

Myth: 'Just Stretch It Out'
Truth: Stretching during an acute spasm activates the stretch reflex, making muscle spindles fire harder. The nervous system interprets this as MORE danger and doubles down on the protective lock. Stretching signals threat, not relief.

Myth: 'Push Through the Pain'
Truth: Movement during acute spasm reinforces the nervous system's emergency response. Each attempt to move triggers more threat detection, creating a vicious cycle. Rest is not weakness, t's the intervention your spinal cord needs.

Seek Medical Attention if you experience:

- Loss of bowel or bladder control
- Progressive leg weakness or numbness
- Saddle anesthesia *(numbness in groin/inner thigh)*
- Fever with back pain

Understanding the Spasm Mechanism

What you're experiencing is the muscle guarding reflex, a protective neuromuscular response controlled by the spinal cord. When the nervous system detects instability or threat, it triggers an involuntary lockdown to prevent further injury.

The Vicious Cycle

Spasm → Ischemia *(reduced blood flow)* → Pain *(waste buildup)* → MORE spasm. This neurological lock bypasses conscious control, you cannot 'stretch it out' or 'breathe through it.'

For Jay,

Thirty years of friendship, steadiness, and a lot of stories. You've been there in the real ways that matter.

Your openness to new ideas and ways of doing things. Your discipline, and the way you never give up on your friends. The dedication you have to your own body, incorporating the breathing and myofascial release into your life. All these traits I admire.

Thank you for your help in design and production of the Backhealer ball and yoga strap set.

Through the years, you have encouraged me to keep going, to think bigger, and to be a better man. I hope I may have done some of this for you.

As iron sharpens iron, so one man strengthens, brightens, clarifies, and steadies the life, presence, and direction of his friend.

Stephen

Author's Note

I didn't invent anything in this book. The breath work has been practiced for thousands of years. Yogis used wooden balls long before I ever touched a Backhealer ball. The movements have been adapted from yoga, exercise therapy, and basic human mechanics.

What I did was pull these pieces together in a way that made sense for my structure, and for those who came to me, because nothing else had worked for them.

I was born with severely degenerated L4-L5 and L5-S1 discs. I've lived with Grade 2 spondylolisthesis my entire life. My spine has been unstable for sixty years. For more than two decades in my Vancouver studio, I've worked with people in every stage of pain. This method wasn't an idea, it was forged through injury, recovery, and years of clinical practice.

I focused on sciatica in this book because the pattern is consistent and the solution is clear. These principles can be applied to almost all back and body conditions.

When the front body changes, when it lengthens, softens, and releases, load shifts off the spine. When load shifts, symptoms often change with it.

This book is for anyone living with pain, recovering from pain, or trying to understand why their body keeps speaking in the same language over and over again. What's in these pages can stand alone or complement any therapeutic work you're already doing.

I offer it with humility and straight truth.

These tools helped me rebuild a body that was never structurally healthy. They can help you rebuild yours.

Stephen

Table of Contents

The secret that changed ME.

Suzannah came home from the seminar *glowing*.

I was on the sofa. My usual spot in those days, managing the constant low-grade pain that had become my baseline. I was somewhere in my forties. I'd been doing yoga for years by then, Bikram mostly. Sweating through 90-minute classes in that brutally hot room, trying to reform a body that had been broken since birth. The yoga helped. It kept me functional. But "functional" and "pain free living" are not the same thing.

"Steve, you have to try this," she said, dropping her yoga bag and mat by the door. "The breathing techniques the instructor shared affect the brain and can actually rewire pain patterns."

Can you believe it?

I nodded politely! But inside I felt that familiar weight settle in my chest. You know, the exhaustion of hope deferred. I'd heard versions of this before. “Try this supplement. Try this therapy. Try this ancient technique.”

I'd tried them all. I'd spent decades in pain, searching for answers in chiropractic offices, doctors' clinics, inversion tables, and ashrams.

Breathing? Just breathing? It seemed too simple. Too soft. Too easy to be the answer to four decades of structural collapse.

But Suzannah wasn't someone who chased fads. She was serious, grounded. And something in the way she described it. The specificity of the technique, the focus on the pelvic floor and diaphragm, the methodical control, made me curious.

Maybe this was a *secret***?**

I set immediately to do what I always do: research.

My close friend and Ayurvedic teacher, Shiva, directed me to B.K.S. Iyengar's “Light on Pranayama”.

Opening that book was like walking into a cathedral. Iyengar didn't treat breath as casual or incidental, he treated it as architecture. He wrote about the pelvic floor as the foundation, the diaphragm as the engine, the ribs as the expanding walls. He described breath not as air moving in and out, but as a tool for nervous system regulation, for fascial release, for reprogramming the medulla oblongata, the primitive brain that governs our pain responses and survival patterns. I read it again and again.

MY FIRST PRANAYAMA PRACTICE

It was mid-day. I was alone on the sofa. AGAIN.

I sat up, placed my hands on my lower ribs the way Iyengar described, and began to breathe through my nose, slowly, deliberately. Engaging my pelvic floor first, feeling it subtly contract and anchor before drawing air down into my lungs. Expanding my ribs in all directions like a balloon. At first, nothing. Just breath. Just me sitting there, wondering if I'd bought into another false promise.

But I kept going. Five minutes. Ten minutes. And then. **Something shifted**. My body began to release. Not the forced relaxation of stretching or heat, but something deeper. My fascia, that dense web of connective tissue that had been locked down for decades, started to soften. My nervous system, which had been in a state of chronic alarm since childhood, began to quiet. I didn't have words for it then, but I was teaching my body that it was safe that **I** was here.

I kept researching. I kept practicing. I made a decision that some thought was extreme, I gave my expensive glass and metal coffee table to my nephew. I put mirrors on the walls of my living room. I laid out my mat, arranged my homemade balls *(small, medium, large)* and I displayed pages from a black and white yoga book on the walls. Beautiful pictures of yogi masters performing the postures that I wanted to learn.

For the next 10 years this is where I transformed.
My lab, my clinic, my dojo.

THOUSANDS OF HOURS

I wasn't training for a marathon or preparing for a competition. I was trying to survive. To function. To reclaim my body from four decades of collapse. On that hardwood floor, I experimented with breath, release, and movement.

It took me two years to work up to a 90-second inhale. Two years of daily practice to develop my pelvic floor, transverse abdominals, and diaphragm to that level.

I used release balls obsessively. I tried every variation - different sizes, different densities. I worked on releasing every muscle/tendon/fascia that felt locked.

Hundreds of movements, hundreds of postures. Such a novice.

In those years it was just me. Me and the floor. Me and the breath. Me and the mirrors showing my alignment, my compensation patterns, my slow, incremental progress.

THE BREAKTHROUGH

It happened one morning, maybe seven or eight years into my practice. Yes, it took me a long time as I did not know what I was doing, and there was little myofascial research available at the time.

Doing my usual psoas/iliacus release (*1st firing hip-flexors*). On my yoga mat. On hardwood. Hard ball pressed deep into the front of my left hip, Nose breathing. Staying present. And then I felt it:

It let go! not just released a little, the PSOAS let go.

The knot that had been there for forty years unraveled. The tissue softened. The tension dissolved.

The constant pulling of the L5 vertebrae *(bottom of spine)* over the sacrum was gone. The intense searing daily pain eliminated.

I stood up, walked to my dresser, and bent forward to put on my socks.

I stopped mid-motion, frozen, not from pain but from disbelief. It didn't hurt. For the first time in forty years I could bend forward without bracing, without fear, without that deep ache in my low back and hips. I put my socks on standing up.

I sat on the edge of my bed and sobbed.

That morning, standing in my bedroom at forty years old, finally touching my toes, I understood what I'd been doing for ten years: I'd been lengthening my front body. The psoas, the iliacus, the diaphragm, all of it had finally released enough for my spine to decompress.

Lengthen the front. Strengthen the back.
A life-changing *secret* **when combined with the breath.**

THE CALLING

I had already been a personal trainer for over 20 years at this point. One of my clients, Eric had sciatica, he was a gastroenterologist. I gave him my handmade psoas ball and taught him the psoas/iliacus release with the breathing.

"Eric," I asked, "please try this for a few days and tell me honestly. Can this cause damage? Can it hurt the colon, the organs, anything in the abdomen?"

A gastroenterologist is a medical doctor who specializes in the diagnosis and treatment of digestive system disorders. They treat conditions affecting the esophagus, stomach, intestines, liver, pancreas, and gallbladder, and perform procedures like endoscopies and colonoscopies.

He came back a week later. "Steve, this might be one of the greatest back pain tools I've ever used. My sciatica is gone."

That was the validation I needed. I could go deeper. I could teach this. I started a small class, a handful of people. Then more. Then more, and then Suzanah taught the first official class. Every time someone stood up after the class and said, **"I haven't felt this good in years,"** I understood. This isn't just for me. This is for everyone.

THE COST

Ten years on that floor cost me almost everything.

Friendships faded. Social invitations stopped coming. Work opportunities passed me by. I missed parties, trips, events.

While others were building careers and families and lives, I was on the floor, breathing, pressing a ball into my hip, watching myself in the mirror doing movement. People thought I was obsessed. Maybe I was. But what they didn't understand, what no one who hasn't lived with this level of chronic pain can understand , is that **I didn't have a choice!**

> **This controlled breath, this directed breath, taught me that pain isn't just structural, it's neurological.**

- It's stored in fascia, in memory, in the primitive brain that governs our fight-or-flight response.
- Pranayama *(breath control)* taught me that the pelvic floor is the foundation of spinal stability, organ support, breath mechanics, even emotional regulation.
- Breath taught me that **you can't force healing.** You can only create the conditions for it. You breathe. **You wait. You listen. You allow.**
- Breath control taught me that the diaphragm and the psoas are connected, literally and functionally, and that when one is tight, the other compensates. When one releases, the other follows.
- Breath taught me that most back pain doesn't start in the back. It starts in the front, in the shortened, collapsed, locked-down front

- body that pulls the spine forward and compresses the nerves from the inside out.
- And breath taught me that if **I could heal myself** this way, I could teach others to heal themselves too.

THE METHOD

Forged in desperation on that living room floor, refined through obsession, and validated by results. First in my own body, then in my clients. Thousands of people who walked into my Vancouver studio and onto my web platform over the years, many of them barely able to move, most of them told by doctors that surgery was their only option.

It's simple and powerful:

Breathe: inhale through your nose, use your pelvic floor and diaphragm to calm your nervous system and create space.

Release: Use sustained myofascial pressure to soften the front-body fascia that's pulling you into collapse.

Strengthen: Rebuild the posterior chain, the back body, so it can support you without strain.

Integrate: Move with awareness, with length, with breath, until the new patterns become automatic.

A WORD ABOUT SELF-CARE

Become active. In a new way. Slowly. Methodically. Begin to create new habits. Retrain your muscles, tendons, fsacia, and nervous system.

Your health professionals see only moments in your story. An appointment, a scan, a report. The real healing is what happens between those visits: how you breathe, how you move, how you think, and how you rebuild. That's the space where self-care lives.

This work strengthens your relationships with professionals. You will learn to feel and understand your body, giving your practitioners better information. Become a participant in your own healing, not simply a patient. Share what you're learning. Most will welcome your initiative.

A f'ckd up spine. Genetics.

L4-L5: seriously degenerated. L5-S1: mostly non-existent. The shock absorbers at the base of the spine that let you bend, twist, lift, run, gone before I took my first breath.

In their place: vertebrae grinding on vertebrae, bone on bone, and spondylolisthesis where one vertebra slips forward over another. Constant sciatica.

That's just the bottom spine.

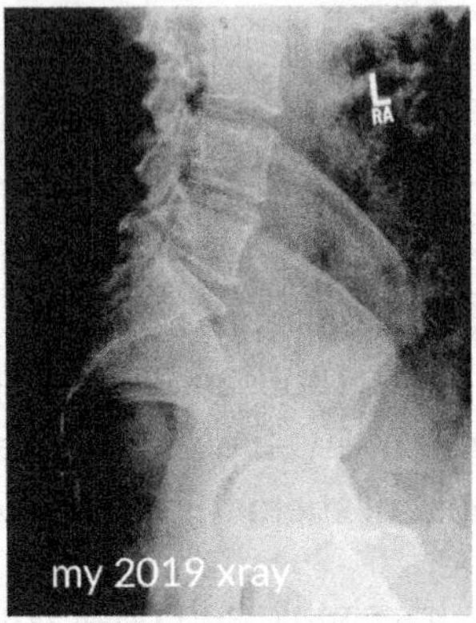

my 2019 xray

Grade 2 *(how far forward one vertebrae is over another)* at birth, and now grade 1. Some structural improvement!

I didn't know any of this as a child, of course. I just knew that my body didn't work right. That I had crushing migraines that would drop me to my knees. That I'd get dizzy and faint for no reason. That something fundamental felt wrong in a way I couldn't articulate.

I started playing hockey when I was young in Toronto, then moved to 100 Mile House, British Columbia when I was seven. A small town. Cold winters. Snow everywhere. And hockey, hockey was my everything.

My favorite team was the Toronto Maple Leafs. Darryl Sittler. Lanny McDonald. Borje Salming. I watched every game. I lived and breathed hockey. It wasn't just a sport, it was my identity, my community, my entire world.

I worked harder than anyone. I built my own ice rink in the backyard, boards, real ice, real nets. Kids from all over the neighborhood would come over to play. It was beautiful.

I trained obsessively. Shot thousands of pucks. Did every drill. Pushed my body to its limits.

But my body had limits I didn't understand when I was young.

THE CONFUSION

We'd do circle drills in practice, skating around the face-off circles, working on crossovers. On one side, I could cross over perfectly. Fast. Smooth. Powerful. On the other side? Nothing. My feet wouldn't cooperate. My body wouldn't generate power. I didn't understand why. None of the coaches understood why. I was strong. I was dedicated. But something in my structure wouldn't allow the movement.

Most of the time, I couldn't get the power out of my body that I wanted. I'd push and push and it was like the signal from my brain got lost somewhere between my spine and my legs. But then once, once, I remember having full power in both legs. Everything connected. I jumped on a loose puck, got a breakaway, and fired it top corner.

I'll never forget that moment, that feeling of full power is unforgettable.

The vertebrae/disc must have aligned perfectly for that one shift. And my body worked the way bodies are supposed to work.

Then that feeling was gone again.

X-RAY AT NINE

My mom, bless her kind soul, drove me an hour each way, once a week, from 100 Mile House to Williams Lake to see a chiropractor. Every week. For years.

I was nine years old when they finally took my first X-ray.

I remember the chiropractor's face when he came back into the room. I could see his concern. **"You have the spine of 150 year old man"** he proclaimed. "You should not be playing hockey, if you get hit the wrong way, **you will be paralyzed**".

This kind man was telling me that the thing I loved most in the world, the thing I did every single day, the thing that defined me, could leave me in a wheelchair.

I quit playing hockey for a year. It didn't make any difference.

The pain didn't stop just because I stopped playing. My body hurt whether I was on the ice or off it. So I thought: If I'm going to be in pain either way, I might as well do what I love.

THE "BUTLER BACK"

I wasn't the first in my family to live like this.

My father had back issues. Bad ones. He had surgery when he was younger, I'm guessing a fusion in the low back, based on the large scar he carried for the rest of his life. He was always in pain. Always. He became an alcoholic. Maybe to cope with the pain. Maybe for other reasons.

But I understand now, as an adult, how chronic pain can drive you to anything that might make it stop, even for a few hours.

We call it "the Butler back." A family curse. A genetic sentence.

My sister had the same surgery my father did. It didn't work. She lived the last fifteen years of her life on the couch, in pain, unable to move, unable to work, unable to live.

I offered to help her. Many times. She refused. I think she'd gotten so deep into the pain spiral that she couldn't imagine a way out. She'd lost hope. And once you lose hope, the couch becomes your entire world.

I'm the one in my lineage who's done the best with this condition. I don't say that with pride, I say it with gratitude.

I just know I couldn't let it win.

THE DAY MY BACK GAVE OUT ON THE HILL

I was in my twenties, working on a ranch. It was also a group home for juvenile delinquents, tough kids, fresh out of prison, and I was responsible for four of them, 24/7. I was fit. I was training. I was still playing hockey at night in a beer league. I was strong.

One day walking up a hill, not a steep hill, just a normal, rolling hill like you'd see on any farm, and BOOM!. Something moved in my low back.

I couldn't walk. I couldn't move. I was frozen in place, and there were people all around me, including the boys I was supposed to be supervising.

They had to get the pickup truck, drive it to where I was standing, and I had to crawl into the front seat on my knees with my upper body draped over the bench seat. That was the only position I could manage.

They drove me back to the main house, not my cabin, because they didn't want the boys to disturb me, and I spent weeks in a room upstairs. I was so embarrassed. Humiliated. Here I was, supposed to be this strong, capable guy working with at-risk youth, and I couldn't even walk up a hill without my spine betraying me.

And this was happening in front of my wife-to-be's family. They owned the ranch. They were watching me lie there, helpless, while their daughter tried to explain that I wasn't weak, I wasn't lazy, I just... had a f'ckd spine.

Nobody understood. How could they? I didn't even fully understand it then, not the way I do now.

All I knew was that I couldn't trust my body. That every single day when I woke up, I didn't know if this would be the day it gave out again. Every movement was a gamble. Every step was a risk. Was I wheelchair bound?

And there was nothing I could do to predict it or prevent it.

That fear, that constant, gnawing fear, was one of the worst parts of living with spinal instability. The pain was terrible, yes. But the uncertainty was suffocating.

THE DAY THE HOCKEY BAG WENT INTO THE DUMPSTER

I was 20, maybe 21. Living in Vancouver. Finished with college. Trying to keep playing, drop-in hockey, beer league, shinny, anything I could find.

But it was getting worse.

Every time I played, I'd be in severe pain for weeks afterward. Couldn't move. Couldn't work. Couldn't function.

Hockey was the only thing I'd ever been good at, the only identity I'd ever had. Until the day I couldn't anymore.

I walked my hockey bag out to the dumpster, gloves, skates, sticks, all my hard-earned, expensive equipment, and I just dumped it in the garbage.

I stood there for a moment. Staring at it sitting on top of the pile. A lifetime of work. A lifetime of identity. A lifetime of me. Gone.

It was heartbreaking. It felt like a death. Because it was, it was the death of the person I thought I was, that I wanted to be. The athlete. The hockey player. The kid with the backyard rink.

I knew, standing there, that things would never be the same. That I'd have to learn to live a life without the thing I'd done every moment of every day since I was a little boy.

DAYS ON THE FLOOR

There have been many, many days and weeks spent on the floor unable to walk. Let me tell you about one of the worst.

This time, I couldn't stand. Couldn't crawl. Couldn't roll over. Couldn't get into the bed. I couldn't take a piss. I couldn't take a shit, though that wasn't usually possible anyway as the colon locks down when the back goes into full spasm.

I was on the floor, on my belly. For three days. Immobile.

Completely on the floor. Not on a mat, not on a bed, on the hardwood floor of my living room. I eventually peed on the floor. I had no choice. After three days, I could crawl. Crawl. Like an infant. And I crawled for another two to three weeks before I could stand and walk again.

That was a very, very dark time. I know some of you have been here as well.

I understand and empathize with you my friends.

THE CAR ACCIDENT

I'm walking, oh, it's about 6:45 in the morning. I'm in the crosswalk, I got the walk signal, I got my coffee in my hand. I am walking back to my studio to train Kate. And all of a sudden I look up, and I think to myself, "oh, this guy driving, he's going to hit me. He's not seeing me. I have the right of way, he doesn't see me."

And then, just at the last moment I jumped the tiniest little bit. Curled into a ball, rolled onto the hood, crushed his hood and windshield with my body. I put a hole in his windshield with my shoulder. Rolled back off the hood, probably tossed me 20 to 30 feet. Rolled onto my knees, did the body scan. I was okay.

The whole time that I was impacting the car, all I could think about was,

my back, my spine, oh, I'm never going to walk again.

He hit me hard. And flung me 30-ish feet. After the body scan, I got over across the street. The paramedics came, and they were like, "wow, you should be dead." They loaded me into the ambulance, took me to VGH, Vancouver General Hospital, emergency. The doctor working that morning, young, nice, very caring. He goes "you got a bruise on your calf where the car hit you. I mean, that seems to be it. "What should we do?" he asked. "Should we CAT scan you?" I replied "I think it's a good idea as who knows, there could be some internal injuries."

He CAT scanned me, and we looked at the pictures together. His face went white "Oh, my God. How are moving around? You really got injured in this accident." I was like, "oh, no, no, no, I've been like that from birth. He states "With your spine you should not be able to walk"

I told him about the breathing, the myofascial release and the movements that I'd been doing for years. And he said, "oh, I'm going to go start doing that right away."

My body's response to this accident was a real witness to all the energy I'd put into it on the floor. I could stand this kind of collision and **I didn't miss a beat**.

SIXTY YEARS OLD

Do I still have episodes? Yes. The discs are still degenerated. The spondylolisthesis is still there. Maybe once a year, my back will lock up enough that I need a few days of intensive self-care, myofascial release, breathing, rest, heat.

But those episodes are different now:

- I can feel them coming. It's not random anymore.
- I know what to do. I'm not helpless, waiting for it to pass.
- They're shorter. Days instead of weeks.
- They're manageable. I don't end up on the floor.
- They don't run my life. I'm not afraid every time I bend over or walk up a hill.

That's what this method gave me, not a perfect spine, but a manageable life. I teach. I demonstrate. I move. I live without the constant fear that defined the first fifty years of my life.

Is that a cure? No. The structure is still damaged. But it's freedom, and after four decades of being a prisoner in my own body, freedom is everything.

Surgery was never an option for me. I dedicated myself to this method and it gave me back my life. **Do it! You will have your life back as well.**

"MIRACLE" BOY

I'm telling you my story not to gain sympathy or to prove I've suffered more than you. I'm telling you this so you understand:

- I know what it feels like to be nine years old and told you might end up paralyzed.
- I know what it feels like to throw away the thing you love most because your body can't handle it anymore.
- I know what it feels like to be strong and fit and still have your back give out on a random Tuesday while walking up a hill.
- I know what it feels like to spend days and weeks on the floor, unable to move, wondering if this time it's permanent.

- I know what it feels like to be told there's no hope, no solution, no way forward.

And I'm here to tell you: There IS a way forward.

But the real proof isn't me. The real proof is Sonnie. He was 13 years old. His mom brought him to me, and he too had a congenital birth defect. His was spondyloptosis, where the L5 vertebrae *(bottom of the spine)* actually sits in front of his sacrum instead of sitting on top of it. I'd never seen this before. I didn't know what to do. I didn't know anything about it. I didn't know if it would work. How did he function? I was so afraid to work with him, to possibly make it worse. But Sonnie would have none of it. He wanted a “normal” life. No he wanted a “super-human” life.

Sonnie learned the breathing, the myofascial release, the movements, and miraculously it worked for him. He is, and was, diligent. He had the worst spine I have ever come across. He carried his myofascial ball with him everywhere to release his spine when he felt it was needed.

A symposium was held at UBC, University of British Columbia. The specialists all attended, There was a gurney on stage for him. Boy were they suprised! He walked up, looked at them. He's 15 years old at this time. Looked at the gurney, **dropped down, did 20 push-ups.**

The specialists were shocked! Kind of upset. They thought Sonnie might have problems in the future with all the parts in the bottom, you know, the genitals and going to the bathroom parts, etc.

Sonnie grew up a strong man. A personal trainer, a yogi, an actor. Still does the method, the Backhealer method. He is healthy, functional, and pain-free.

Sonnie, “MIRACLE BOY”, one of my heroes!

WHAT THIS MEANS FOR YOU

If you have sciatica, a disc bulge/herniation, tight hip flexors, a shortened front body, and a nervous system stuck in protection mode? You might become completely pain-free. Do you have severe structural damage like mine and Sonnies. You might still have occasional episodes, but they'll be manageable. Predictable. Short. And in between, you'll have a life.

Secret **is, no matter whats happening in your spine, in your body, you can heal, you can live a more functional, pain-free life.**

This method, I called “Backhealer”. We are the healers. We apply the method to our backs and bodies. We heal.

The method came from desperation, from necessity, from a refusal to accept that "this is just how it is."

This method gave me my life back.

You can heal. Maybe dramatically. Maybe completely. Maybe just enough to get your life back.

That's what I'm sharing, not false hope, but real possibility.

The body you have today, even if it's damaged, even if it's been in pain for decades, still has capacity you haven't accessed yet.

Now let me show you ***WHY this method it works.***

The practical science

In this chapter we need to discuss just enough science and its application so the mind can better direct your body's healing abilities. For complete research documentation and citations:

OUR FORWARD-BENDING SOCIETY

Take a walk through any city. What do you see? Teenagers shambling down the sidewalk, necks craned forward, shoulders rounded, thumbs scrolling. Like extras from The Walking Dead, except the zombie apocalypse is Tik Tok.

Office workers hunched over laptops, heads jutting forward, chests collapsed, breathing shallow. Eight hours. Ten hours. Twelve hours. Drivers gripping steering wheels, shoulders rotated inward, hands turned palm-down for so long the position feels permanent.

Elderly people bent at the waist, shuffling forward, unable to straighten even if they wanted to. The question isn't "why are they bent?" The question is: "How long have they been ***practicing that position***?"

We are a forward-bending species.

Not just because of modern life, though phones and computers have accelerated the collapse. But because of design. Everything we do is in front of us. Picking things up. Using tools. Working. Eating. Writing. Typing. Driving. Scrolling.

Your hands don't work behind your body. They work in front of you. And when your hands are in front of you for hours every day, your shoulders roll forward. Your chest collapses. Your arms rotate inward, palms turn down, thumbs turn in. Your upper back rounds. Your head creeps forward to see the screen, the phone, the road.

And then there's sitting.

Sitting collapses your hip flexors. Your knees are bent. Your hips are flexed. Hour after hour. Year after year. Until the shortened position becomes your structure.

The front of your body, from below your pubic bone to your collarbones, compresses. Tightens. Shortens. Rotates inward. The lumbar spine responds by moving forward. Do you feel like your belly sticks out sometimes? But you know you are not fat.

> **Could the muscles deep in the front of your spine have shortened so much that you can no longer stand straight without effort? Even sitting is uncomfortable. Standing for long periods of time... forget about it.**

Imagine wearing a tight jacket that's two sizes too small. The fabric pulls across your chest, rounds your shoulders forward, restricts your breathing. You can't fully expand. You can't stand up straight. Every time you try to open up, the jacket pulls you back into collapse. You've been wearing this jacket for 20 years. 30 years. 40 years. And the fabric has fused to your body. It's not clothing anymore, it's your fascia, your muscle, your structure.

That's what chronic anterior chain compression feels like.

And here's the insidious part: your posterior chain *(back, neck, hamstrings, glutes)* has been fighting this forward pull every single day. Trying to hold you upright against gravity. Trying to keep you from collapsing completely into that bent-forward position.

The muscles of your back are exhausted.

They've developed trigger points. They're inflamed. They're tight from overwork, not from being short. And every time they try to pull you upright, the anterior chain yanks you forward again. It's a losing battle. **And then there's the gravity.** Your head weighs 10-12 pounds when it's balanced over your shoulders. For every inch your head creeps forward the effective load on your spine increases by approximately 10 pounds. As you are reading this your head is probably 2-3 inches forward especially if you are reading on a screen.

Two inches forward? You're carrying an extra 20 pounds. Three inches? An extra 30 pounds. All day. Every day. For years.

Your posterior chain *(back body)* is fighting three forces at once:

- The anterior *(front)* pull yanking you forward into collapse
- Gravity constantly pulling you down
- The multiplied weight of your forward head making everything exponentially harder

So when you strengthen your back, when you release your hamstrings, when you get adjusted, you're helping the exhausted side. The losing side. The side that's already overstretched and overwhelmed. The over-worked side, the dominant side, the side creating the collapse and compressing your sciatic nerve, is in the front. That's what needs to release. The anterior chain. ***Imagine finally taking off your compression jacket.***

THE FRONT BODY. THE “ANTERIOR” CHAIN

When I say "front body" or "anterior chain," I mean everything below and in front of your pubic bone all the way to your chin:

- **Hip-flexors:** psoas, iliacus, rectus femoris, the muscles that lift your knee toward your chest
- **Abdominal wall and fascia:** the entire front container of your torso
- **Diaphragm:** your primary breathing muscle, attaching to your spine at L1-L3
- **Chest and shoulders:** pectorals, anterior deltoids, platysma, the upper body muscles that round you forward

These structures work together. When they're chronically shortened and tight, they create a forward collapse pattern that your posterior chain can't overcome, no matter how strong it is, no matter how much you release it. And when they pull your pelvis into anterior *(front)* tilt and your lumbar spine into hyperextension, they compress the nerve roots at L4-L5-S1 that form your sciatic nerve. So even if you don't have structural spine issues you can still experience sciatica.

THE COMPRESSION CYCLE MAY CAUSE SCIATICA

Here's a familiar pattern behind chronic sciatica, and most back and body pain:

Stage 1: You Sit
You sit at a desk. You drive. You watch TV. You sleep curled up. For hours. For years. Your hip flexors stay in a shortened position. Hip flexed. Knees bent. At first, it's just position. But over time, the muscle fibers reorganize. They physically become shorter. The fascia surrounding them thickens. What started as temporary positioning becomes structural adaptation. Scientists call this **adaptive shortening**. After decades of sitting, your psoas isn't just tight. It's short.

Stage 2: Your Pelvis Tilts Forward
When your hip flexors shorten, they pull your pelvis into anterior tilt. The top of your pelvis tips forward, your tailbone sticks out, your lumbar spine hyperextends.

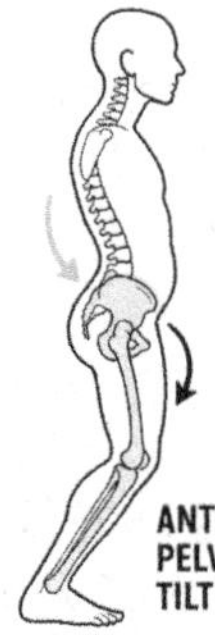

This is where sciatic nerve compression starts.

Your spinal cord runs through your vertebrae. At each level, nerve roots exit through openings called foramina. When your spine hyperextends, those openings get smaller. L4-L5-S1. The nerve roots that form the sciatic nerve. Getting squeezed. Meanwhile, your discs get compressed on the back side and stretched on the front. This is the setup for herniation. But it's not the disc's fault. The disc is just responding to the forces being applied to it.

Stage 3: Your Diaphragm Locks
Your diaphragm is a dome-shaped muscle below your lungs. When you breathe in, it should descend, flatten out, push your organs down and forward, allow your lungs to fill. But the diaphragm attaches to your spine at L1-L3. Right next to the psoas. When the psoas is chronically short and tight, the diaphragm can't descend properly. It gets restricted. Your breathing becomes shallow, chest-dominated instead of diaphragmatic. **The psoas and diaphragm are connected, structurally and functionally. When one is restricted, the other can't work properly.**

Stage 4: Your Nervous System Protects

Your body has a sophisticated threat detection system. When joints are compressed, when nerves are irritated, when breathing is restricted, your nervous system interprets this as danger. It does what it's designed to do: protect. It cranks up muscle tone in your back, trying to stabilize a spine being pulled out of alignment. It creates guarding, protective muscle spasm, around the irritated area. It amplifies pain signals traveling down your sciatic nerve. You experience this as tightness. Spasm. Burning tension. Pain shooting down your leg into your calf or foot. But it's not injury. It's protection. The problem is, it's protecting against a threat that won't go away until you address the root cause.

Stage 5: The Loop Locks In

This goes on for months. Years. Decades. Your nervous system stays in high alert. Your back muscles never rest, they're firing constantly, trying to pull you upright against the forward collapse. They develop trigger points. They become inflamed. They fatigue. And over time, something worse happens: your nervous system becomes sensitized. Normal movements start triggering pain. Light touch feels sharp. The volume knob on your pain system gets turned up, and suddenly even activities that shouldn't hurt, like bending to tie your shoes, create intense symptoms down your leg. Scientists call this **central sensitization**. Pain that started as a mechanical problem becomes a neurological one.

You cannot stretch your way out of this. You cannot strengthen your way out of this. *You have to release the front first.*

FASCIA, THE COMMUNICATION NETWORK

Sciatica is not just about nerves and muscles. There's a third, more secretive, often overlooked player, our fascia.

Fascia is a three-dimensional web of connective tissue that wraps everything in your body. Every muscle. Every organ. Every nerve. Every blood vessel. It's one continuous structure from head to toe. Think of the white membrane you see when you peel an orange, that thin layer between skin and fruit. That's fascia. Except in your body, it's everywhere.

Layered. Interconnected. Communicating.

Fascia provides structure, allows movement, transmits force, and communicates. The layers glide over each other when you move. When fascia is healthy, it's supple, hydrated, and mobile. But when you sit for years, when you're chronically stressed, when you live in protective patterns, fascia changes.

Fascia is made of collagen fibers suspended in a gel-like substance called ground substance. This gel changes consistency based on how you use your body. When fascia is healthy, the ground substance is fluid. The collagen fibers are organized. The layers glide. But when fascia is chronically compressed or immobile, the ground substance becomes viscous, thicker, stickier. The collagen fibers become disorganized, tangled. Adhesions form between layers that should glide independently.

This is densification.

Dense fascia doesn't glide. It restricts. It pulls. It creates tension patterns that radiate far beyond the local area. Dense fascia can create the same symptoms as structural irregularities, nerve compression, or joint dysfunction. You might think your psoas muscle is tight. But often, it's the fascial sheath surrounding the psoas that's dense and restricted. The muscle is stuck inside a container that won't let it lengthen.

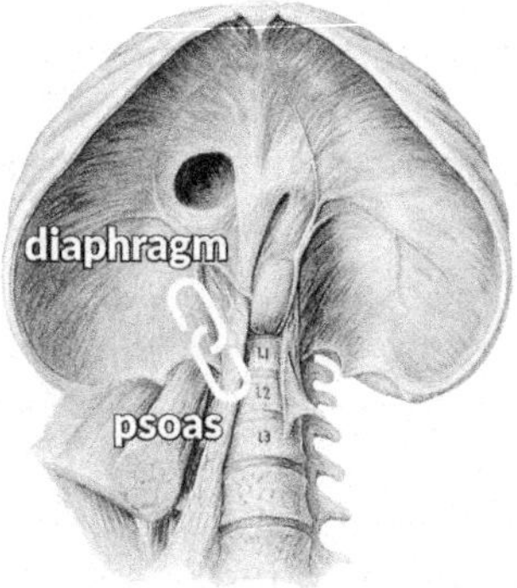

The psoas and diaphragm aren't just neighbors. They're wrapped in continuous fascial sheaths that blend together at the thoracolumbar junction. This fascial continuity means: When your psoas is short and dense, it physically restricts diaphragm descent. When your diaphragm can't move, it creates tension that propagates into the psoas. They literally cannot function independently. This is why you can't just "release the psoas" without addressing breathing. And why you can't restore diaphragmatic breathing without releasing the psoas. **They're part of the same system.**

FASCIA RELEASES WITH SUSTAINED PRESSURE

When you apply sustained pressure to dense fascia, combined with slow breathing and small movements, several things happen:

- **Mechanical deformation:** The pressure physically creates space between the layers
- **Piezoelectric effect:** Fascia responds to mechanical pressure by becoming more hydrated at a cellular level
- **Thixotropy:** The ground substance changes from gel to liquid state under sustained pressure, allowing the fibers to reorganize
- **Mechanoreceptor activation:** Pressure activates sensory nerve endings that signal the nervous system to reduce protective muscle tone
- **Heat generation:** Sustained compression combined with breath creates local temperature increase, enhancing tissue pliability

This isn't massage. This isn't stretching. This is sustained, intelligent pressure that gives fascia time to reorganize. When it works, you feel it, **that "melt" sensation**. The tissue softening. The layers starting to glide. Space opening where there had been compression. The fascia is reorganizing.

Fascia is continuous.
Releasing the psoas affects the diaphragm.
Releasing the diaphragm affects the ribcage.
Releasing the ribcage affects the shoulders.
It's all connected.

IS THE BREATHING REALLY THAT IMPORTANT?

Mechanically:
Deep diaphragmatic breathing creates pressure changes in your abdomen and thorax. This rhythmic pumping moves fluid through your fascia. The connective tissue needs fluid circulation to stay supple. When you breathe shallowly, this pump doesn't work. Fascia becomes dehydrated. Sticky. Dense. When you breathe deeply and slowly, you're literally hydrating your tissues. Making them pliable. Capable of change.

Neurologically:
Breathing has many roles, we focus primarily on two.

1. Inhaling through your nose, stills your mind, and takes your patterned brain "off line", so you can create new pain and movement patterns.
2. Exhaling through your mouth slowly, activates your vagus nerve, the main nerve of your parasympathetic *(rest and heal)* system. Heart rate slows. Blood pressure drops slightly. Stress hormones decrease. Inflammatory markers reduce. Muscle tone globally decreases.

Measurable. Reproducible. Real.

The difference is profound. After controlled breathing, tissue that was resistant becomes responsive. Guarding drops away. The nervous system allows release. Without the breath work first, the body stays in protection mode. <u>No amount of pressure gets past that defense.</u>

TISSUE RESTRUCTURING TAKES TIME

Minutes to Hours: Immediate Relief
When you apply sustained pressure with slow breathing, something changes immediately. The tissue softens. You can move more easily immediately. Pain decreases. This is ***thixotropy***, fascia becoming more liquid under sustained pressure. But this change is temporary. Without continued practice, the tissue returns to its dense state.

Days to Weeks: Nervous System Reprogramming
After a few weeks of daily practice, changes last longer. Movement patterns that used to trigger sciatica start feeling safe. This is your nervous system ***updating its internal map***. When you've had chronic pain, your body schema gets distorted. Movements that should be safe get flagged as dangerous. Areas that should move freely get locked down. But when you practice and repeat conscious pain-free movement your brain revises its predictions. "This movement doesn't hurt. Maybe it's not dangerous." The protective response down-regulates. Muscles that were constantly firing learn to relax. Amplified pain signals diminish.
This takes weeks. Around week 4-6, you notice: mornings are less stiff, transitions are smoother, **the leg pain quiets down.**

Weeks to Months: Structural Remodeling
The deepest changes take months. Fascia and tendon don't just stretch. They remodel. The cells that build connective tissue detect the new mechanical loads you're applying. They break down old, disorganized tissue and lay down new, aligned tissue. Collagen fibers reorganize. Dense adhesions dissolve. Atrophied muscles rebuild. This is biological remodeling. It cannot be rushed.

- Muscle hypertrophies in 2-4 weeks.
- Tendon takes 6-12 weeks.
- Bone takes 3-6 months.
- Fascia sits in between. Around month 6, something fundamental shifts.

Changes aren't just lasting, they're compounding. Each week better than the last. The sciatica that used to flare with every wrong move becomes less reactive. Capacity builds. Function returns.

Months to Years: Consolidation
Eventually, the new patterns become automatic. You're not "managing" sciatica anymore. You're living. Your nervous system rewrites its motor programs. Your tissues restructure. The front-body compression pattern releases. The structure may still show disc bulges on MRI. But the forces acting on that structure have changed completely.

REMEMBER SONNIE? "MIRACLE BOY"

Scan 100 people with zero leg pain, people who've never had sciatica, who run and hike and live normally, and 30-90% will have disc bulges and herniations at L4-L5 and L5-S1 *(lowest vertebrae where the sciatic nerve emerges)* on their MRI. ***Sonnie? Spondyloptosis? He defies the laws of physics.***

One of the most liberating discoveries came from working with **David. 58. Engineer. Chronic sciatica for 12 years**. MRI showed disc bulges at L4-L5 and L5-S1, facet arthritis, spinal stenosis. Tremendous pain down his leg into his calf. His orthopedic surgeon recommended fusion surgery. He came to me as a last attempt before surgery. We worked together for three months. Breathing. Myofascial release. Movement retraining. Daily practice, no exceptions. His sciatica decreased by 70%. He could return to normal function. Play with his grandkids. Walk without fear. David went back to his surgeon for follow-up. They did another MRI. The surgeon called me, "What did you do? His imaging looks the same. The bulges are still there. The stenosis hasn't changed. **But his pain is gone. How?"**

HOW? BODIES DISTRIBUTE LOAD DIFFERENTLY

Two people with identical disc bulges: one has chronic sciatica, one runs marathons. Why?

The pain-free person's mind and body have learned to distribute forces through their hips, through their thoracic spine, through a diaphragm that actually moves. The damaged segment isn't taking all the stress. The person in pain has compensatory patterns, tight hip flexors, restricted breathing, fear-avoidance, central sensitization, that focus all stress on the already-compromised segment.

Sciatica *secret* **! Structure and pain <u>do not correlate</u>.**

This was revolutionary for me. It means your structure doesn't define capacity. It means disc bulges aren't a death sentence. It means you can optimize function even when structure is damaged. That's what we did for David. We didn't fix his discs. We taught his body to move better, breathe better, distribute forces better. The damaged segments were still there, but they weren't being overloaded anymore.

WHAT "RESEARCH" ACTUALLY SHOWS

The Diaphragm-Psoas Connection

Turkish researchers recruited 60 people with chronic low back pain. Half received standard physical therapy, ultrasound, hot packs, generic exercises. ***The other half received diaphragm and iliopsoas myofascial release(MR)*** combined with the same generic exercises.

After 4 weeks the myofascial release group saw **pain drop by 60%** *(from 6.8/10 to 2.7/10)* The standard therapy group saw pain drop by only 20% The MFR group **gained three times more flexibility and breathing capacity.**

Motor Control Training:

A major review analyzed 29 studies involving over 2,400 people with chronic low back pain. Key findings:

- Conscious motor control exercises reduced pain by 10-15 points on a 100-point scale at 3 months (general exercise: only 5-8 points)
- Disability improved by 5-10 points (general exercise: 2-4 points)
- Benefits persisted at 12 months
- Particularly effective for people with poor movement patterns and segmental instability

Breathing Training:

A systematic review examined 15 studies with over 700 participants **using just controlled breathing for chronic pain.**

Findings:

- Pain intensity reduced by 22-35% after 4-8 weeks
- Heart rate variability improved by 15-30%—indicating better autonomic regulation
- Effects were dose-dependent: more practice = better outcomes

Another study tested controlled breathing in people with chronic low back pain. Results after 4 weeks:

- **Pain dropped** from 6.2/10 to 4.1/10 (**34%** reduction)
- Catastrophizing decreased 28%
- **Muscle tension** decreased **32%**

Pain Neuroscience Education:

Damage does not equal pain. MRI findings don't define capacity. This isn't just philosophy, acquring knowledge has measurable effects.

A review of 17 studies with over 1,000 people showed:

- Immediate pain reduction: 14 points on a 100-point scale (control: 7 points)
- Disability improvement: 10 points (control: 3 points)

- Fear-avoidance beliefs dropped 20%, critical because fear-avoidance is a stronger predictor of disability than actual tissue damage

Combined Approaches:
When you integrate multiple components, education, breathing, tissue release, motor control, effects compound.

A major overview analyzing 264 studies with over 21,000 participants found multicomponent interventions (exercise + education + self-management) showed substantially superior outcomes to single interventions.

Another review of 41 trials with nearly 7,000 people showed integrated approaches produced moderate-to-large effects, with nearly double the odds of return to work compared to usual care.

Different components target different systems. Combining them produces additive or synergistic effects.

MY CLINICAL REALITY

While each component has solid research support, the specific integration I teach, breath-coupled anterior myofascial release followed by progressive motor control, hasn't been tested in large randomized trials. What I can tell you from 25 years in my Vancouver studio, working with thousands of clients with sciatica:

Approximate outcomes:

- 80% experienced significant improvement (≥75% pain reduction, return to stopped activities)
- 15% experienced moderate improvement (40-60% pain reduction, some functional gains)
- 5% experienced minimal improvement (often those who couldn't commit to daily practice or had complex additional health problems)

Timeline to meaningful improvement:

- Weeks 1-4: Noticeable changes (breathing easier, morning stiffness reduced, leg pain quieter)
- Weeks 5-12: Functional improvements (walking without limping, sitting without flare-ups, bending without fear)

- Months 3-6: Substantial capacity increases (returning to sports, traveling without worry, living normally)

Likely outcome (70-80% probability):

- Significant pain reduction in your leg and calf
- Functional improvement (return to stopped activities)
- Possibly occasional flare-ups (but you'll know how to handle them)

Timeline:

- Weeks 1-4: Nervous system changes, breathing improves, pain intensity decreases
- Weeks 5-12: Tissue remodeling begins, motor patterns encoding, sciatica becomes less reactive
- Months 3-6: Capacity building, return to activities, confidence restoration
- Months 6-12: Consolidation, maintenance, occasional tune-ups

THE HONEST BOTTOM LINE

This method is structurally sound, evidence-informed, clinically tested, and honestly presented.

- **Anterior chain release works**
- **Breathing retrains your nervous system**
- **Fascia responds to sustained pressure**
- **Conscious motor control beats general exercise**
- **Pain education changes outcomes**
- **Progressive exposure reverses sensitization**
- **Integration is more powerful than single interventions**

The solution is simpler than you think: Lengthen the Front, Strengthen the Back. Release what's pulling your spine into compression, then rebuild what's been exhausted from compensating.

A little more science in the next chapter, before we get to the practice.

"Lightning bolt" down your leg

The first time it happened to me, really happened, I was 10 years old, reaching down to pick up a hockey stick. Not lifting anything heavy. Not twisting awkwardly. Just bending forward to grab a stick off the ice. This electric current shot from my lower back, through my left buttock, down the back of my thigh, past my knee, all the way to my foot. Like someone had plugged me into a wall socket.

I dropped to one knee. Couldn't breathe for a second. And when I finally stood up, my left leg felt... wrong. Numb in some places, on fire in others, and weak in a way I'd never experienced.

That's sciatica.

You probably know that feeling. Maybe yours came on gradually. Maybe it hit you like mine did, sudden and shocking. Either way, you know that electric quality. That shooting, searing pain that follows a specific path down your leg. Here's the *secret* I wish someone had told me back then: **sciatica isn't a diagnosis. It's a symptom.**

Calling your leg pain "sciatica" is like calling your fever "thermometer syndrome." The fever is real, but it's telling you something else is going on. The same is true for sciatica. Understanding what's actually happening, and more importantly, what's NOT happening, changed everything for me.

WHAT SCIATICA TRULY IS

Our sciatic nerve is the longest and thickest nerve in your body. It starts in your lower back, specifically from nerve roots at L4, L5, S1, S2, and S3, and runs through your buttock, down the back of your leg, all the way to your foot. When we talk about sciatica, we're describing pain that follows this nerve's pathway.

The pain typically:

- Shoots down one leg (rarely both at the same time)
- Follows a predictable pathway, what anatomists call a dermatome

- Feels electric, burning, or like lightning bolts
- Comes with tingling, numbness, or that "pins and needles" feeling
- Usually feels worse than any back pain you might have
- Gets triggered by specific movements, sitting, coughing, bending forward

There's a clinical test called the straight leg raise. If lying on your back and lifting your straight leg reproduces that shooting pain, it's a strong sign of nerve root irritation.

THE TWO PART ATTACK

Doctors told me that my structural problems would cause sciatica for life. They were half right. Yes, I had structural issues. Yes, those issues created the conditions for nerve irritation. But what they missed, what almost everyone misses, is that sciatica involves two actions happening simutaneously. **Mechanical compression** AND **chemical irritation**.

Mechanical Compression:
Something is physically touching or pressing on your sciatic nerve. In about 90% of cases, it's a bulged/herniated disc. The soft, gel-like center *(nucleus pulposus)* pushes out through the tough outer layer and ends up right where your nerve root exits the spine. This most commonly happens at L4-L5 or L5-S1, the two lowest discs that bear the most stress.

But here's what's crucial: it's not just the disc pushing out. It's what's pulling your spine into a position where the disc has no choice but to bulge/herniate. The anterior chain compression you learned about in Chapter 3, that's what creates this setup.

Chemical Irritation:
This is what nobody told me for decades, and it's why sciatica can be so intense. When disc material leaks out, your body treats it like a foreign invader. It triggers a massive inflammatory response that floods the area. These chemicals directly attack the nerve. **They're caustic. Irritating.**

So you're not just dealing with physical pressure. **You're dealing with a chemical assault.** That's why sciatica feels different from other pain. It's not just "something's pressing on me." ***It's "I'm being attacked."***

While **disc bulge/herniation** causes most sciatica, I've also seen it from:

Spinal stenosis: the spinal canal narrows and pinches nerve roots.

Spondylolisthesis: one vertebra slides forward on another

Degenerative changes: bone spurs or arthritic changes reducing nerve space

Piriformis syndrome: the piriformis muscle in your buttock compresses the sciatic nerve.

Your shortened front body is pulling your spine into positions that trap the sciatic nerve. Lengthen the front. Free the nerve.

THE SCIATICA TIMELINE

Sciatica at day 3 is completely different from sciatica at week 12, which is completely different from sciatica that's been around for two years. Understanding where YOU are changes everything about how you approach it.

Acute Sciatica (Less than 6 weeks)

What it looks like:

- Recent onset, often from a specific incident
- Intense inflammation, that chemical assault is at its peak
- Usually from disc herniation with acute inflammatory response
- The most dramatic symptoms, but ironically, the best prognosis

80-90% of acute sciatica cases resolve within 6-12 weeks.

What you need:

- Calm the inflammatory response
- Maintain tolerable movement *(not bed rest, not aggressive exercise)*
- Start the breath work immediately
- Don't let fear take root, this isn't permanent

Subacute Sciatica (6-12 weeks)

What it looks like: You're past the initial crisis, but it's not resolving as fast as you hoped. Symptoms might be improving slowly, or they've plateaued. You're starting to wonder if this is your new normal.

What you need:

- Progressive neural mobilization
- Conscious motor control retraining
- Address fear-avoidance before it becomes habit
- Patient persistence with the work

If symptoms are gradually improving, keep going. If they're worsening or you're developing new neurological deficits, that's when we consider imaging.

Chronic Sciatica (Beyond 12 weeks)

What it looks like:

- Symptoms persisting well beyond typical healing timeline
- Often multifactorial, not just the original disc herniation anymore
- Central sensitization has developed *(nervous system oversensitivity)*
- Psychological and behavioral factors are now significant players

What you need: Everything in this book, the breath work, the releases, the movement retraining. Understanding you're not broken, your system is stuck in a protective pattern.

Chronic sciatica is not a life sentence. I had it for decades. Told it was permanent. What actually guaranteed it was the anterior chain compression pattern I hadn't addressed. Once I released that pattern, the chronic sciatica resolved. Not because the structure changed. Because the forces acting on that structure changed.

WHEN YOU NEED TO SEE A DOCTOR IMMEDIATELY

I'm all for self-care. This entire book is about taking control of your own healing. But there are times when sciatica isn't just sciatica.

Cauda Equina Syndrome (Medical Emergency)
This is rare, but it's the one that terrifies every spine specialist.

Go to the emergency room immediately if you have:

- **Loss of bowel or bladder control *(not just difficulty, but actual incontinence)***
- **Numbness in the "saddle" area *(groin, inner thighs, buttocks)***
- **Progressive weakness in BOTH legs**
- **Sexual dysfunction that came on suddenly**

Don't wait. Don't call anyone. Don't try the ball work. Call 911 or go to the ER. This requires emergency surgery. Hours matter.

Other Red Flags

- Progressive motor weakness: Numbness and tingling aren't an emergency. But significant, worsening weakness, especially foot drop, needs evaluation.
- Signs of infection or tumor: Fever, unexplained weight loss, night sweats, or unrelenting pain that doesn't respond to ANY position changes.
- High-risk history: Previous cancer, significant trauma, or immunosuppression with new sciatica needs imaging to rule out serious pathology.

5 MYTHS THAT KEEP YOU STUCK

Myth 1: It's Permanent Damage

The truth: 80-90% of acute sciatica resolves naturally as your body reabsorbs disc material. I've had clients with "massive disc extrusions" on MRI, convinced their life was over, who six months later showed complete reabsorption on follow-up imaging. Your structure might not change. Mine didn't. But the forces acting on that structure can absolutely change.

Myth 2: The Size Predicts the Pain

You can have a massive disc herniation with minimal symptoms. Or a tiny bulge creating excruciating pain. Studies show 30-40% of people with absolutely no back pain have significant disc abnormalities on MRI. Your pain-free neighbor might have a herniation that would make your radiologist wince.

What matters more:

- Exact location relative to the nerve root
- Chemical inflammatory factors
- Nervous system sensitivity
- Anterior chain compression

I've worked with clients whose MRI showed "minimal disc changes" but who couldn't stand upright. Why? Because their psoas was so tight it pulled their entire spine into a position that irritated the nerve root.

Myth 3: Movement Equals Damage

This one kept me prisoner for years. I thought: if movement triggers the pain, movement must be damaging something. So I avoided anything that might "aggravate" it. This led to progressive deconditioning, fear-avoidance behaviors, muscle atrophy, and loss of confidence. The truth: Yes, there's a time for relative rest in acute, severe sciatica. That time is measured in days, not months. Conscious strategic movement is what heals, not protective stillness.

Myth 4: It's the Same as General Leg Pain

True sciatica:	**Referred pain from tight muscles:**
Follows a specific nerve pathway	Diffuse, achy, or cramping
Sharp, electric, or burning quality	Doesn't follow a nerve pattern
Shoots or radiates in a line	Often stays in buttock or posterior thigh
Numbness or tingling/specific areas	No true neurological symptoms

This distinction matters for treatment approach.

Myth 5: You Have a "Bad" Disc

This language drives me crazy. "Bad disc." "Damaged spine." You don't have bad body parts. Well, you might. But mostly you have inflammation around a nerve root responding to stress it couldn't adapt to in that moment. If you sprain your ankle, you don't have a "bad ankle." You have a temporary inflammatory response to tissue stress. Your ankle went through more demand than it was prepared for. The same is true for your disc. Your disc experienced more mechanical stress than it could handle. Now you have inflammation. That's not the same as permanent damage or defectiveness.

I was told I had a "degenerated spine" at 9 years old. I did and still do. That I'd be in a wheelchair by 30. That my body was failing. My body was responding predictably to abnormal mechanical forces. I changed those forces, and everything changed. The force/load on your body needs to change. *Secret.*

THE MIND GAME

When there is a lightning bolt of pain shooting down your leg, your brain makes a reasonable conclusion: Something is seriously wrong. I need to protect this. Movement equals danger. This triggers guarding, bracing, avoidance, hypervigilance, and catastrophic thoughts about the future. This fear response becomes the problem.

I watched a client, Sarah, a 48-year-old dancer, with a disc herniation at L5-S1 that looked terrible on MRI. The radiologist used words like "severe, significant impingement", and "you are not 20 any more maybe your dancing career is over."

She refused to accept his warnings. So she did the work. The breath. The releases. The movement retraining. Her pain decreased inversely to her fear. As she became more confident, as she moved more boldly, as she stopped treating herself like she was broken, she got better.

Her follow-up MRI? The herniation was still there. Hadn't changed much.

But **she was dancing again.**

Your nervous system takes cues from your interpretation of danger. If you treat every twinge as tissue damage, your nervous system amplifies its protective response. Pain increases. Movement decreases. Sensitivity heightens. This doesn't mean your pain is "all in your head." Your pain is real. The nerve irritation is real. The inflammation is real. But your response to it, your beliefs about what it means, your behavioral adaptations, your expectations about your future, these shape whether it resolves or becomes chronic.

Matter follows mind!

Maybe your sciatica stems from your shoulder

Her name was Jessica. She came to me with left-sided sciatica that had been constant for six months. Electric pain down her left leg. Numbness in her left foot. Classic presentation.

She'd done everything. Physical therapy focused on her left side. Chiropractor adjusting her left hip. Massage therapist working her left piriformis. Nothing helped.

Jessica laid on my table for assessment. On her back. I checked her psoas, her iliacus, her hip flexor, all on the left side where the pain was. Everything was tight. Everything needed work. But something looked... off.

I had her stand up and look at herself in the mirror. "What do you see?" I asked. "I don't know. Just me?" "Look at your shoulders." She looked. Paused. "My right shoulder is higher. And more forward."

"Now look at your hips." Another pause. "My left hip looks... higher?" "Exactly. Your right shoulder is pulling forward and up. Your left hip is hiking in response. And your spine is twisted between them like a wrung-out towel."

"But my pain is on my left side. My left leg." "I know. But I think your left-sided sciatica is the RESULT of your right shoulder pulling against your left hip. Your body is twisted three-dimensionally. And that twist is creating the compression that's irritating your nerve."

She looked skeptical. "So... you're going to work on my right side? The side that doesn't hurt?" "Exactly." I got to work on the right upper torso. I did not work on the "painful" left side.

When she stood up, she said, "My leg feels... different. Less electric. More quiet"

Two weeks of working diagonally, right shoulder, left hip, balancing both sides, and her left-sided **sciatica was 80% better.**

That's when I fully understood, the body doesn't just collapse forward and back. **It collapses in a spiral**. And if we only address the front-to-back compression, we're missing half the picture. **Another** *secret*?

BEYOND FRONT AND BACK: THE MISSING DIMENSION

Your body doesn't exist in only two dimensions. You're not a flat cardboard cutout. You're a three-dimensional structure that moves in rotation, that twists, that spirals. When your body collapses, when years of sitting, stress, and compensation patterns take their toll, it doesn't just fold straight forward.

Your body spirals as it folds.

Look at yourself in a mirror right now. Really look. Feet together. Is one shoulder higher than the other? Does one shoulder sit further forward? Does your head tilt slightly to one side? Does one hip appear higher or more forward than the other?

Most people have asymmetry. And that asymmetry isn't random, it's a pattern. A rotational pattern that creates diagonal lines of tension through your entire body. This is the three-dimensional reality of collapse, you're not just folding forward, you're spiraling as you fold. This spiral, this rotation, is often what's creating your sciatica.

Your Body's Spiral System: The Diagonal Slings

Your shoulders and pelvis are connected by diagonal fascial lines that run through your torso like suspension cables on a bridge. When your right shoulder rotates forward, your left hip compensates. When your left shoulder elevates, your right hip drops. The spine twists between them, creating torque, compression, and, often, nerve irritation along the sciatic pathway. There are two main diagonal slings:

The Anterior Oblique Sling
This runs from your abdominal muscles on one side, across your body through the fascia, to the opposite hip flexor.

Example: **Your right side connects diagonally to your left hip.**

When this diagonal line shortens, from sitting twisted toward your computer screen, or always carrying a bag on one shoulder, it creates rotational tension through your entire torso. Your right side pulls forward and down. Your left hip compensates by pulling up and back. Your spine twists between them. Suddenly you have left-sided sciatica that no amount of stretching will fix.

The Posterior Oblique Sling

This runs from your back muscles on one side, through the lower back fascia, to the opposite glute.

Example: Your left upper back connects diagonally to your right glute. When this sling is imbalanced, when your left upper back is tight and your right glute is weak, you get rotational instability in your pelvis. Your body compensates by over-tightening other structures. And often, that compensation creates sciatic nerve compression.

When one diagonal dominates, you get torsion through your spine, asymmetric loading on your discs, and one-sided pain patterns. And often, that sciatica is on the OPPOSITE side from where the primary problem lives.

COMMON ROTATIONAL PATTERNS

Pattern 1: The Desk Worker Spiral

- Right shoulder forward and elevated (from mousing)
- Left hip hiked and tight *(compensating)*
- Head tilted slightly right
- Spine rotated to the right

Result: Often creates left-sided sciatica

Why? The right shoulder pulls the diagonal sling that crosses to the left hip. The left hip hikes to stabilize. This creates compression on the left L5-S1 nerve root.

The Pain Trap: You focus on your left side, stretching the left hip, massaging the left glute. But the driver is on your RIGHT side. Until you release the right shoulder and chest, the left hip will stay compensated and the sciatica will persist.

Pattern 2: The Driver's Twist

- Left shoulder elevated (resting on the door/window)
- Right hip compressed (from gas/brake pedal position)
- Torso rotated slightly left
- Right psoas chronically shortened (from pressing pedals)

Result: Often creates right-sided sciatica

Why? Hours in the car create a locked rotational pattern. Your left shoulder pulls up, your right hip compresses down, and your spine twists between them.

The Pain Trap: You try to stretch your right hip or strengthen your right glute. But the pattern is maintained by the elevated left shoulder and the rotational habit. You have to address the whole spiral.

Pattern 3: The Phone Caller Collapse

- Both shoulders rounded forward *(from looking down at phone)*
- Head jutted forward *(tech neck)*
- One hip higher than the other *(usually the dominant side)*
- Overall forward collapse with rotational component

Result: Can create bilateral sciatica or alternating sides

Why? The forward collapse is present, but it's not symmetric. One side bears more load than the other. Symptoms might switch sides depending on what you did that day.

The Pain rap: Symptoms alternate, you think it's just "general instability." But it's asymmetric front-body collapse with rotational loading. You need to address both the forward compression AND the rotational pattern.

SELF-ASSESSMENT: FIND YOUR PATTERN

Test 1: The Mirror Test

Stand in front of a full-length mirror wearing minimal clothing.

Look at your shoulders: Is one higher than the other? Does one sit further forward?

Look at your hips: Is one hip bone higher than the other? Does one hip appear to sit further forward?

Look at your head: Does it tilt to one side? Does it jut forward? Is it centered over your pelvis, or shifted?

What this tells you: If you see clear asymmetry *(most people do)*, you have a rotational pattern.

Test 2: The Rotation Test

Stand with your feet hip-width apart. Arms relaxed at your sides. Don't move your feet or knees. Rotate your torso to the right as far as you comfortably can. Notice how far you can turn. Rotate your torso to the left as far as you comfortably can.

Compare the two sides: Can you rotate equally in both directions? Is one side significantly more restricted? Does rotating toward one side reproduce or increase your sciatica symptoms?

What this tells you: If one direction is notably more restricted, your fascia has adapted to a rotational pattern. If rotation reproduces your leg symptoms, rotation is definitely part of your sciatica pattern.

Test 3: The Cross-Body Shoulder Test

Sit or stand comfortably. Bring your right arm across your body *(like you're giving yourself a hug)*. Use your left hand to gently pull your right elbow further across. Feel the stretch in the back of your right shoulder. Hold for 10 seconds. Bring your left arm across your body. Use your right hand to gently pull your left elbow across. Feel the stretch in the back of your left shoulder. Hold for 10 seconds.is probably tighter. This cross-body relationship is your diagonal sling at work.

Compare the two sides:

Is one shoulder significantly tighter? Does stretching one side change your sciatica symptoms (better or worse)?

What this tells you: The tighter shoulder is often on the OPPOSITE side from your sciatica. If you have left sciatica, your right shoulder

THE THREE-DIMENSIONAL SCIATICA TRUTH

Jessica's left-sided sciatica came from her right shoulder. Your sciatica might be the same, an echo of an upper-lower imbalance, a diagonal compensation pattern that's been locked into your fascia for years.

This is why treating locally often fails. You're chasing the pain instead of addressing the pattern.

The method I'm about to teach you addresses all three dimensions: front-to-back compression, diagonal patterns, and rotational imbalances. It's all connected. It's all one system.

The remainder of the book will teach specific techniques that lengthened my front body, strengthened my back body, decompressed my nerve roots, and **gave me my life back** after decades of sciatica.

David got his life back.

Jessica got her life back.

Sonnie got his life back.

Join us.

The method, Backhealer

The Core Principle

Lengthen the Front, Strengthen the Back

That's it. That's the method. The front body *secret* from Chapter 3 wasn't just a discovery, it's the entire approach.

How the Method Works

The Backhealer is synergistic. All elements work together simultaneously:

Breath integrates into everything. You breathe during myofascial release work. You breathe during movement. Easy nose breathing becomes your new normal, shifting your nervous system from threat to safety.

Lengthen the front through myofascial release. Ball work on psoas, iliacus, diaphragm, chest, and diagonal slings creates space and releases fascial restriction.

Strengthen the back as you create length. As your anterior chain releases, your posterior chain must strengthen to hold this new position against gravity. Release creates space for strength. Strength maintains release.

This happens simultaneously, not in stages.

What You Need

The Backhealer Ball (or same size softball, *the sport*)
Purple ball for the core front-body releases. I'll explain the ball design in the Resources section.

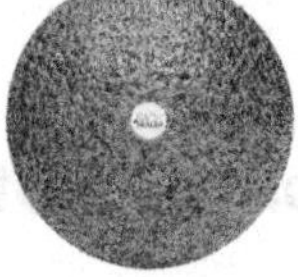

Your Mat or Carpet
A dedicated mat for your practice. This mat becomes your healing space.

Heat
Practice in a warm environment. Heat makes fascia more pliable. Turn up the heat, use a space heater, or practice after a hot bath/shower.

Your Sacred Space
Place your mat somewhere you won't be disturbed. The same spot every day. **Your nervous system responds to ritual and consistency.**

Consider adding:

- **Scent:** I burn incense before every session. The smell signals my body: it's time to let go. You might use essential oils or a candle.
- **Soft lighting:** Not bright lights. A lamp or candles that signal this time is different.

Use the same space daily. The same mat. The same time if possible. Your body learns: **when I come here, I release.** This isn't superstition. This is neurology. Consistent cues create consistent responses. **Your dojo!**

Time Commitment
This method works, but it requires practice, especially in the first 8-12 weeks. Timing below is approximate.

- Weeks 1-6: 15-30 minutes daily - Breathing integrated with myofascial release, and M1 movements
- Weeks 6-12: 30-45 minutes, 4-5 times per week - Breathing integrated with myofascial release, and M2 movements
- 12 weeks and after: 30+ minutes, as needed - Add M3 movements if they feel good. Listen to your body, you'll discover which releases and movements work best for you. **Consider keeping a journal to track your healing process.**

GO SLOOOOOOW

Here's what I need you to understand: it's better to do too little than too much, especially in the first six weeks. Your mind and body need to accept what you're about to do. This work is powerful. You might not believe that breathing and ball pressure can be life-changing, but it is. I've seen it thousands of times. I've lived it myself. You might be sore the first few days and weeks. Like the soreness you get when you start going to the gym. That's normal. That's your body waking up.

But don't push through it. Don't try to force results.

As a trainer, I learned that people go too quickly trying to produce results when the body takes a minimum of six weeks to learn and re-pattern new movements.

Your internal map, your body schema, needs time to reorganize. This timeline also depends on your current health and any other complications you're dealing with.

Start where you are. Make it work for your body.
If psoas release is unavailable to you, if it's too intense, too hard to lay on your stomach, if your body says no. Start with chest and shoulder release on a wall or door frame. Start there. Build from there.

It took me awhile to get used to this work too. The intensity. The slowness. The waiting. Now I crave it. My body knows: this is how I heal. This is how I stay free.

Trust your breathing. It tells you how your nervous system is responding to what you're doing. If you can breathe into it, you have permission to stay with it. If you're holding your breath, back off. Listen. Adjust. Try again tomorrow.

Go sloooooow. Be patient. Let your body learn.

GOOD PAIN VS BAD PAIN

Good Pain (Therapeutic Discomfort):

- Your breathing is always under your control. Inhaling through the nose. If you hold your breath, your body has gone into fight or flight.
- Deep, achy, intense pressure
- "Hurts so good" sensation, uncomfortable but somehow right
- Makes you breathe DEEPER, not hold your breath
- You can feel tissue yielding, softening, "melting"
- You can stay with it, settle into it
- Might make you emotional (tears, sighs, releases), that's okay
- Feels like something is opening, releasing
- Your body says "yes, this" even though it's intense

Bad Pain (Stop Signal):

- Your breathing is NOT under your control. Breath holding.
- Sharp, stabbing, electric
- Shoots down your leg *(reproduces your sciatica)*
- Makes you automatically tense, brace, guard
- Your whole body screams "GET OFF"
- Feels like damage is happening
- Increases your symptoms after you're done

The Test:
Can you keep breathing slowly and deeply? = Good pain, keep going
Do you automatically hold your breath? = Bad pain, back off

The Rule:
Work at 6-7 out of 10 intensity. Not 9-10 *(heroic suffering doesn't release fascia, it just traumatizes tissue)*. Not 3-4 *(too gentle, nothing happens)*. The sweet spot is where it's intense but breathable.

The Principle:
Your nervous system knows the difference between therapeutic work and threat. If you can breathe into it, you have permission to stay with it. If your body says NO, if you're bracing, guarding, holding your breath, listen. Back off. Find a gentler entry point. Take load off your ball or back out of the movement.

This work is not about toughing it out. It's about intelligent pressure and movement combined with breath. Force doesn't release fascia. Patience does.

Tissue takes time.

HOW IT WORKS, MARCUS'S STORY

Marcus came to me with sciatica that had been constant for three years. He, like Jessica, had done everything. Physical therapy, chiropractic, acupuncture, massage, epidural injections. Nothing worked for him. His MRI showed a disc herniation at L5-S1. The first session, I had him lie on his back and breathe for 10 minutes. Slow, controlled nostril breathing.

He thought I was crazy. "I need my disc fixed," he said. "What's breathing going to do?"

After 10 minutes, his body softened slightly. His ribs were moving. His belly wasn't rock-hard anymore. His nervous system was beginning to shift from threat to safety. His back flattened out.

He rolled over and I placed the ball under his psoas, about two inches to the right of his navel and two inches down. Right where the psoas crosses over the pelvic brim. He immediately came off the ball. Not from pain, but from the intensity of the sensation.

"That's not my back," he said. "Why does pressing on my stomach make my leg stop hurting?" Because his psoas, that deep hip flexor running from his lumbar spine to his leg, was pulling his vertebrae into a position that compressed his L5 nerve root. His disc herniation was real, but it was the end result of years of this pulling force.

"That's... intense," he said. "Is it pain or pressure?" I asked. "Pressure. Deep pressure. Like you're pushing on something that hasn't been touched in years."

“That's exactly right. Now breathe into it. Slow balloon breath. Fill your belly around the ball." He inhaled. His belly expanded. The ball pressed deeper into the tissue. "Now exhale. Long, slow exhale. Let everything soften."

As he exhaled, "I felt it," he said as the tissue yielded. “Just slightly. A millimeter of give where there had been none.” We held that point for three minutes. **Just breathing. Just allowing.**

"How's your leg?" I asked. He paused. "The burning... it's less. The electricity is still there, but it's not as sharp."

We moved to three more points along his psoas. Each one, the same process: find the spot, breathe into it, hold for three to five minutes, allow the release.

Twenty minutes of work. Four points. Just breathing and sustained pressure.

When he stood up, he moved differently. His pelvis wasn't tilted forward anymore. His spine had length. His right leg, the one that had been on fire for three years, **felt quiet.**

"It's not gone," he said. "But it's... different. Like the volume got turned down."

Six weeks of daily practice, breathing integrated with myofascial release and conscious movement, and Marcus's sciatica resolved completely. Not because his disc magically healed, although that will happen as pressure is released. Because the fascial tension pulling on his spine released, and the mechanical compression on his nerve root stopped.

That's what you're about to learn. Where to place the ball. How to breathe with the pressure. How to recognize release. Then how to create new patterns of breath and movement.

The same work that freed Marcus. The same work that freed me.

Let's begin with the breath, pranayama.

Control the breath, control the mind.

Control the mind, control the body.

Breath, your healing engine

Breathing is simple. Automatic. Boring, even. Something your body just does without you having to think about it. Breathing is automatic. Your brainstem controls it, keeping you alive even when you sleep. But there is a difference between **breathing to survive and breathing to heal.**

Most chronic pain sufferers breathe poorly. They breathe shallowly, using their chest and neck muscles instead of their diaphragm. They breathe quickly, maintaining a constant state of low-level stress in their nervous system. Many are mouth-breathers.

This dysfunctional breathing pattern maintains pain.

Breath is fundamental to your healing. I spent the first two years of my practice learning to breathe properly for this reason. This single practice may be the most powerful tool you ever learn.

Every meditation tradition, Buddhist, Hindu, Taoist, Sufi, Christian creation, has breath at its core. Not from superstition, but from an understanding that breath is the bridge between body and mind, conscious and unconscious, suffering and healing.

Control your breath, and you control your nervous system. Control your nervous system, and you control your pain. This is the engine of the entire system.

WHY THE BREATHING *(PRANA)* NEEDS TO BE CONTROLLED *(YAMA)*

Uncontrolled breathing, automatic, unconscious, directionless, cannot resolve chronic pain. Here's why: Modern posture compresses the front body. Forward-bent posture from sitting, driving, screens shortens the psoas, compresses the diaphragm, and collapses the chest. This compression reduces blood flow, lymphatic drainage, and interstitial fluid movement. Compression traps metabolic waste. When tissue can't circulate fluid properly, metabolic by-products accumulate. Lactic acid, inflammatory markers, cellular debris, these pain-generating substances

substances have no pathway out. They sit in the tissue, triggering pain signals continuously.

Automatic breathing can't solve this. Your brainstem keeps you alive, but it doesn't direct healing. Automatic breathing maintains the status quo. It doesn't increase regional blood flow. It doesn't create pressure gradients to clear waste. It doesn't tell your autonomic system to shift from stress to safety.

The director *(mind)* must show the way. **Pain has a door**, the circulatory and lymphatic systems. But without conscious direction, that door stays closed. The mind must activate the breath engine, then guide it to the compressed tissue.

- Then blood flow increases at least 13%.
- Then waste clears.
- Then the autonomic system recognizes safety and releases guarding.

This is why breath must be controlled. Not "better" breathing. Controlled breathing. **Intentional. Directed.** The mind initiates. The brain executes. The mind returns to guide. The brain delivers the physiology. Without this sequence, pain has nowhere to go.

HOW MIND AND BRAIN WORK TOGETHER

The breath amplifies healing when the mind and the brain work together in the correct sequence.

Step One: Mind Initiates

Healing begins with the mind, not the brain. The mind makes the decision to practice pranayama. You choose to fire the pelvic floor, the diaphragm, and the transverse abdominis with precision. You choose to control the inhale and lengthen the exhale. You choose to engage the breath deliberately rather than automatically. This is conscious intention. This initiates the practice.

Step Two: Brain Executes

Once the mind initiates the pattern, the brain takes over the mechanics. Not imagination; this is brain cortical activation. The motor cortex fires the diaphragm. The phrenic nucleus at C3-5 sends signals through the phrenic nerve. The pre-Bötzinger group in the medulla coordinates the rhythm. The somatosensory cortex maps the sensation. The interoceptive networks in the insula track internal body states.

When you practice correctly, these circuits strengthen, refine, and accelerate. Neural pathways become myelinated. Firing patterns become automatic. **The breath becomes an engine.**

WHAT THE ENGINE CREATES

- The descending diaphragm stretches the vena cava, increasing venous return from the abdomen to the heart.
- Four ligaments connecting the pericardium to the diaphragm create negative intrathoracic pressure, a vacuum effect that pulls blood upward and increases cardiac filling
- Pressure shifts
- Circulation increases
- Fascial hydration improves
- Autonomic tone moves toward parasympathetic dominance
- The nervous system recognizes safety

This is the difference between living on autopilot and activating your potential.

Step Three: Mind Returns to Direct

Now the engine is running, stronger, clearer, and more powerful than passive breathing could ever produce. At this moment, the mind reenters the process.

The mind says to the brain, in effect:

- You've built the pressure.
- You've coordinated the muscles.
- You've activated the engine.
- **Now send this energy here.**

This is where intention directs physiology.

THE SCIENCE OF DIRECTED ENERGY

When the mind guides the breath toward a specific area, a joint, an organ, a fascial plane, a region of tension, the brain responds automatically. The brain maps your body topographically in the somatosensory cortex of your brain. When you focus attention on your psoas, neural activity increases in the specific cortical region that represents your psoas. That increased neural activity triggers local blood vessel dilation in that body region.

Blood flow, volume, and oxygenation increase by up to 13%. This is called neurovascular coupling. It's measurable with PET scans and fMRI.

When attention combines with the pressurized breath engine:

- **Neural activity increases in the corresponding cortical map**
- **Blood vessels in that region dilate**
- **Circulation increases 13% or more**
- **Oxygen delivery increases**
- **Metabolic waste clears more efficiently**
- **Fascia absorbs and releases fluid**
- **Protective guarding reflexes soften**

The mind guides the brain. The brain delivers the blood flow. The tissue responds.

The Sequence
This is the "magic" of intention and breath working together.

1. **Mind initiates the breath**
2. **Brain executes the pranayama mechanics**
3. **Mind returns to guide where the engine works**
4. **Brain delivers the physiology (13% increase in regional blood flow, oxygen, waste clearance)**

Breath is the engine.
The brain powers the engine.
The mind steers it.

THE ANATOMY THAT MAKES IT WORK

The Diaphragm: Your Primary Breathing Muscle

TOP

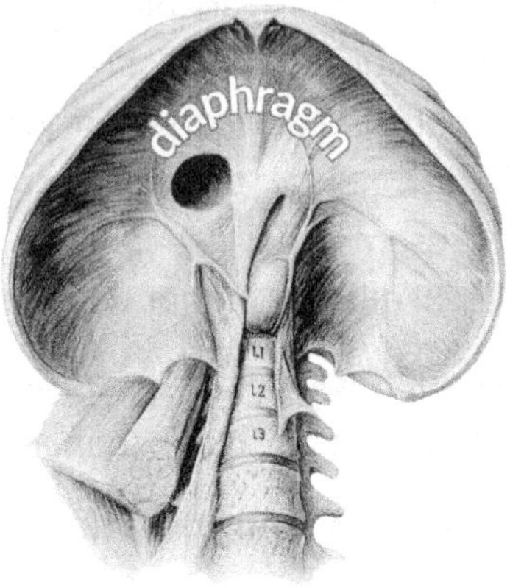

The diaphragm is a dome-shaped muscle below your lungs, separating chest and abdominal cavities. It attaches to the lower ribs all around, and its crura anchor to the lumbar spine at L1–L3, adjacent to the psoas.

This is not coincidental. The diaphragm and psoas are intimately connected through fascia, shared vertebral attachments, and function.

On a proper inhalation, the diaphragm contracts and descends toward the pelvis. This creates a vacuum in the chest cavity that draws air into the lungs. Draws, not pushes. On exhalation, the diaphragm relaxes and rises, the ribs soften inward, and air flows out.

The Pelvic Floor: The Foundation of Breath

As we gently contract the pelvic floor muscles we create a base for pull and support.

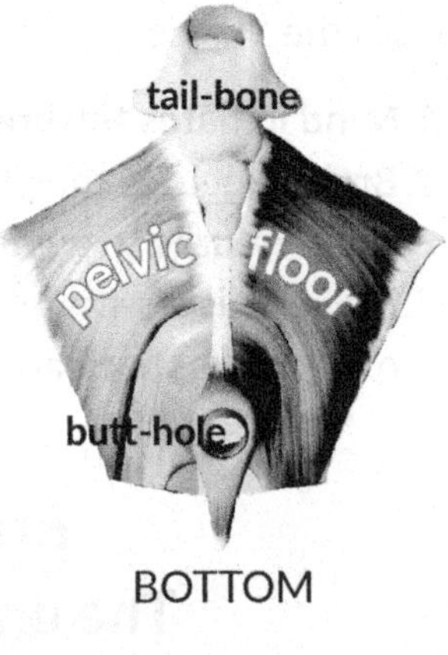

BOTTOM

The pelvic floor is the hammock of muscles at the base of the pelvis, the levator ani, coccygeus, and associated fascia. It supports organs, stabilizes the pelvis, and coordinates with every breath.

The pelvic floor has two layers. The deep layer provides core stability; the superficial layer assists with sphincter control. Both layers must engage properly for therapeutic breathing.

Where is it exactly? It is the muscles around your butthole.

If you have chronic pain, your pelvic floor doesn't work properly.

Prolonged sitting, chronic guarding, anterior pelvic tilt, and shallow breathing all contribute to pelvic floor dysfunction: weakness, poor engagement, delayed activation, and poor endurance.

The Diaphragm–Psoas–Pelvic Floor Triad

The diaphragm, psoas, and pelvic floor function as one integrated system.

Think of a container:

- Diaphragm is the lid (TOP)
- Pelvic floor is the base (BOTTOM)
- Transverse abdominis is the wall (sides)
- Psoas links spine and pelvis through the center

When this system coordinates, you get true core stability, efficient breathing, and internal spinal support. When one element fails, the others compensate. A tight, elevated diaphragm undermines pelvic floor function; a weak pelvic floor limits diaphragmatic descent; a shortened psoas restricts both.

This is why you start with breath work. Until the diaphragm moves properly, nothing else works optimally.

THE PRACTICE OF BREATH CONTROL *(PRANAYAMA)*

This is already simplified from traditional Iyengar teaching. If you want the full classical method, study with a qualified teacher. What I present here is the therapeutic application, the mechanics you need for pain relief and fascial release.

Setup: Lie on your back with knees bent and gently together, feet flat. Or sit up comfortably. One hand on chest, one on belly. Eyes closed if comfortable.

Step 1: Awareness
Notice current breathing without judgment, chest or belly, nose or mouth, fast or slow.

Step 2: Nose Breathing *(Non-Negotiable)*

Mouth closed. Inhale and exhale through your nose. Nasal breathing calms the system and conditions air. If you're breathing through your mouth, close it. This is foundational. If emotion releases during practice, you may exhale through the mouth briefly, then return to nasal breathing.

Step 3: Engage the Foundation *(Pelvic Floor and Transverse Abdominis)*

Build the foundation.

Before inhaling, gently engage your pelvic floor muscles. Contract inward with subtle downward energy toward the feet. Think of the base of a dome gently flattening, creating about 20-30% engagement. At the same moment, draw the deep abdominal wall (transverse abdominis) in and down toward the spine. The belly does not pouch passively; it is contained and supportive.

Step 4: Inhale *(Diaphragm Descends, low ribs draw in, upper ribs expand)*

Maintain both foundation engagements as air is drawn in.

The diaphragm contracts and descends like a piston. The downward pull of the pelvic floor and inward draw of the transverse abdominis create an anchor below. This assists diaphragmatic descent above, amplifying the chest vacuum and drawing air in with less effort.

The upper ribs expand circumferentially, sides and back, to create true 360-degree expansion.

The expansion happens in the ribs, not the belly. The belly moves toward the spine as the transverse abdominis engages; the lower ribs move inward as the diaphragm descends. The chest fills last and least. The hand on your chest moves minimally; the lower ribs widen noticeably. Allow the breath to be drawn in by the vacuum you have created.

This is not passive. The downward engagement of pelvic floor and inward draw of transverse abdominis create an anchor/base. The diaphragm and ribs contract using this base to enable strong oppositional forces. This is not weak chest lifting. Your thoracic cavity is expanding like a balloon.

If your shoulders are lifting and your chest is the primary mover, stop. Focus on downward pull from the bottom and back. Keep shoulders quiet.

The Balloon Visualization

As you inhale, visualize your lungs and ribs as an elastic balloon. The balloon fills from the bottom up:

- Pelvic floor is the base of the balloon
- Diaphragm descends, balloon begins to inflate
- Lower ribs expand circumferentially - sides and back
- Upper ribs fill last
- The balloon gets bigger and bigger with each inhale

Breath Counting: The Mental Focal Point

Count silently during each phase of breath:

- Inhale: 1... 2... 3... 4... (one count per second)
- Pause at top: 1
- Exhale: 1... 2... 3... 4... 5... 6... (exhale as long as needed)
- Pause at bottom: 1

The counting focuses your mind on a focal point so youur mind cannot wander.

Progression: Start with a 4-count inhale, 6-count exhale. As your capacity grows over weeks and months, your counts will extend:

Step 5: Pause at the Top

Pause briefly at the top of the inhale, count "1 and" to acknowledge fullness, then begin the exhale. Do not clamp or hold tension. Just recognize the transition. This is not a long, tension-filled breath hold. J**ust a brief acknowledgment**, "1 and" . No straining.

Step 6: Exhale Completely

Begin a slow nasal exhale. The cascade reverses: ribs soften inward, diaphragm rises, transverse abdominis releases, pelvic floor returns to resting position. **Try exhaling past your usual stopping point.** Allow the ribs to draw in more than normal, the belly to flatten, and the natural compressive action of the core to press out the last air. **Do not force or strain**; simply finish the breath.

Why the **complete exhale** matters:

- **Cleansing effect.** You release not only carbon dioxide but metabolic by-products that accumulate in chronically contracted tissue as lymph and venous flow improve with pressure changes.
- **Elasticity.** Taking the lungs and rib cage through full range builds pliability and capacity.
- **Enhanced next inhale.** A true empty sets up a stronger vacuum for a fuller, easier inhalation.

Visualize the release: As you exhale, see waste, stale tension, and old holding patterns leaving. Imagine dark heaviness moving up and out through the nose. You are clearing space.

- Chest tightness: sternum, intercostals, and anterior chest fascia
- Any restriction: place a hand there and breathe into that space

Step 7: Pause at the Bottom

At the bottom of a complete exhale, pause for "1 and." This empty space often carries primal anxiety. Do not rush. Teach the nervous system that emptiness is safe and the next breath always arrives. Repeat: Pause briefly at both transitions, top and bottom, then begin again: pelvic floor and transverse abdominis engage, inhale; complete exhale; brief pause.

Practice for seven minutes when you are first learning. Not two. Not five. 7 full minutes.

What You Should Feel

- Belly stays relatively flat or draws slightly inward on inhale
- Lower ribs expand to the sides and back
- Neck and shoulders remain quiet
- Mind settles after a few minutes
- A felt sense of mastery and calm emerges

If you feel like you're forcing, straining, or your jaw is clenching, back off. This is controlled power, not force. Strong yet unhurried engagements. You are strengthening your breathing muscles with every practice. Go slooooow.

USING YOUR BREATH ENGINE

The seven-minute practice trains the breath. It builds the neural pathway, strengthens the pelvic floor, and teaches your nervous system the pattern. But you do not breathe this way constantly.

Think of pranayama as a pump, or an engine that you turn on when you need it. Once activated, the pump moves energy, shifts alignment, resets your nervous system, and opens restricted tissue. Then you can return to natural breathing.

When to activate the pump:

- At the beginning of every session
- During practice: Brief activation to set proper alignment or reset when you feel compensation patterns emerging
- When pain arises: several focused breaths directed into the area
- When energy drops: a few strong cycles to pump fresh energy up the spine and restore alertness
- To change alignment: engage the foundation, breathe, feel your position reorganize

Between these activations, breathe naturally through your nose. Easy, relaxed, efficient breathing. You are not performing pranayama every second of every session. The pump primes the system. Natural breathing maintains it.

A Warning, Sort Of

Practice daily and you may feel **"superhuman"** in the only way that matters: actual control over your autonomic state and a reliable path to transform pain through breath.

Master this engine and everything else becomes possible.

Myofascial release for sciatica

Sciatica is nerve compression at three primary sites: the lumbar spine where nerve roots exit at L4-L5-S1, the pelvic outlet where the nerve passes through the pelvis, and the deep hip where it travels beneath the piriformis. One-sided sciatica often mirrors one-sided chest collapse, creating a diagonal fascial pull from shoulder to opposite hip.

These four releases decompress the sciatic nerve at each entrapment point.

- **The psoas restores length to the front body and decompresses the lumbar nerve roots.**
- **The iliacus opens the pelvic outlet.**
- **The chest release corrects the diagonal pattern.**
- **The piriformis frees the final bottleneck in the deep hip.**

Address the front body and the nerve has space to heal.

Before You Begin: Essential Preparation

- Empty your bladder. You will be applying pressure to the lower abdomen.
- Wait after eating. Two hours after a large meal; one hour after a light one.
- Create your space. Firm surface, warm quiet room, no interruptions.
- Keep tools nearby. Balls. Pillows, blankets, and one to three books for ball elevation.

Ball Selection - see Resources for more detail.

Use the purple ball *(softball size)* for psoas and iliacus release on the floor. Elevate on books for deeper reach if needed. Also use for chest and shoulders on door frame or wall. Use the green ball *(baseball size)* for deeper glute, piriformis, and hip-rotator work. Avoid textured balls, they irritate fascia. If improvising, wrap a regulation softball/baseball in thin carpet foam and smooth tape. Never use lacrosse or wooden balls on the abdomen, they are too hard and trigger guarding. Balls not rollers, as they cannot penetrate.

A. RELEASE YOUR PSOAS MUSCLE

When the psoas shortens and hardens, it pulls the lumbar spine into hyperlordosis, compressing the nerve roots at L4-L5-S1 where the sciatic nerve begins. This is the primary compression point for most sciatica.

A shortened and hardened psoas muscle can:

- Tilt the pelvis forward, altering hip-joint geometry and closing the pelvic outlet through which the nerve passes
- Restrict the diaphragm, keeping the nervous system in low-grade fight-or-flight
- Force the back muscles to overwork until they spasm and fatigue
- Shut down glute activation, weakening hip support

Release the psoas and the entire body begins to reorganize.

What. Where. The Psoas Muscle.

The psoas major arises from the sides of T12 through L5 and the intervertebral discs between them, passes through the pelvis, and inserts on the lesser trochanter *(inside of leg, 2–3 inches below pubic bone)* of the femur.

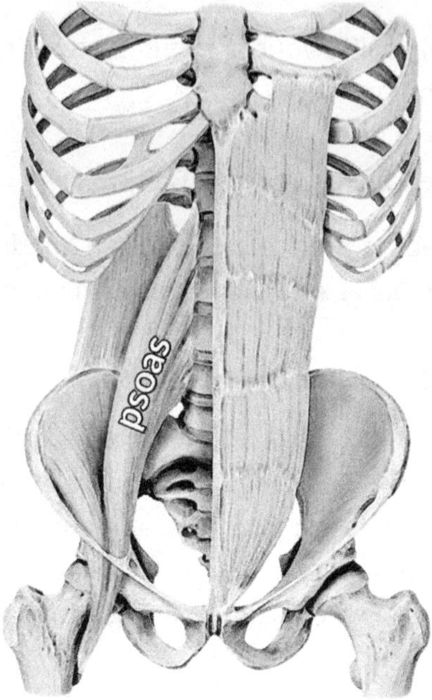

It acts both as first-firing hip flexor and as a deep stabilizer of the spine, coordinating with the diaphragm and pelvic floor. It lies behind the abdominal organs and peritoneum, accessible through sustained pressure with the ball and breath.

Safety Guidelines for All Releases

Stop immediately if you experience:

- Sharp, electric, or shooting pain
- Nausea
- Inability to breathe fully
- Progressive weakness, numbness, or loss of bowel/bladder control

For nerve pain that shoots below the knee, move the ball a half-inch to shift off the nerve itself. For pain directly on bone, adjust position slightly to move into the soft tissue corridor.

The Release Sequence and Positioning

Step 1: Activate the Engine *(Before Placing the Ball)*

Lie in position. Perform 3-5 full pranayama breaths:

- Foundation engages *(pelvic floor and transverse abdominis)*
- Balloon fills from bottom to top
- Ribs expand 360 degrees
- Count: 1-2-3-4 on inhale, 1-2-3-4-5-6 on exhale

This shifts your nervous system from stress to safety. The engine is now running.

Step 2: Position the Ball

Place it precisely on the landmark. Let your weight settle gradually onto the ball. Exact positioning is coming next.

Step 3: Direct the Breath

Now the mind returns to direct. With each exhale, guide the breath into the tissue under the ball. This is where vessels dilate, oxygen rises, waste clears, fascia hydrates, and guarding releases. Visualize the balloon filling, then emptying directly into the tissue under pressure. Each exhale softens the tissue from rock to clay.

Step 4: Count and Sustain

Continue counting each breath: 1-2-3-4 inhale, and exhale slowly. The counting focuses your mind. With this focal point, the mind cannot wander. Around breath 8-10, the nervous system recognizes safety. The tissue begins to release.

What to Maintain During the Hold

- Continuous nasal breathing. Never hold your breath
- Each exhale directed into the ball. Mind guides the breath to the tissue
- Balloon visualization - See the elastic balloon filling from bottom to top, then emptying into the compressed tissue
- Count every inhale breath - This keeps your mind focused and present

Detailed Ball Positions for Psoas Release

Locating the starting point: from the ASIS *(front hip bone)* move approximately 2 inches toward midline and 1–2 inches down. The soft corridor between ASIS and navel is your target.

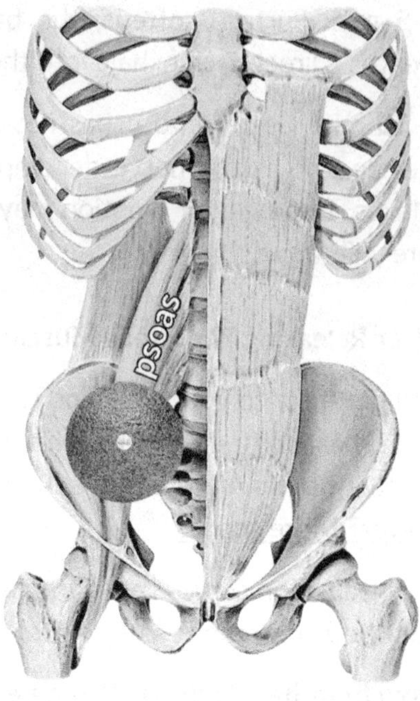

For sciatica: Start with your pain side. After 15 minutes, assess your symptoms. If pain has reduced significantly, you're done for today. If not, release the other side.

<u>Position 1</u>: Face Down on the floor or bed *(Primary)*
Place the **purple ball** on that point; elevate on 1–3 books if needed. Legs extended behind you or same-side leg slightly bent. Arms beside you or on forearms. Keep pelvis neutral.

Adjusting Pressure:

- More: Straighten legs, relax completely, sink weight onto ball
- Less: Prop on forearms, bend knees, reduce book height

Position 2: Side-Lying *(Alternative)*

Lie on your side with the ball under the same landmark. Bottom leg straight or slightly bent, top leg bent forward for control. Roll your weight slowly onto the ball.

Position 3: Seated *(Modified)*

Sit on the edge of a firm chair, place the ball between the lower abdomen and chair back, and lean in. Less effective but accessible for limited mobility.

What You May Feel

0–1 min: Broad pressure, tenderness, thickness. Activate the breath engine—3-5 full pranayama breaths to shift into parasympathetic.

1–5 min: Surface softens; the ball begins to sink. Continue counting breaths. Direct each exhale into the tissue under the ball.

5–20 min: Getter into psoas now. Warmth or tingling may travel down the leg, this is the nerve decompressing. Sensation eases; whole body relaxes. Trembling or emotion may surface, allow it. Your nervous system is recalibrating.

After Releasing The Psoas Muscle

Roll gently onto your back and rest for 2-3 minutes. Let the floor tell you what has shifted. Breathe softly through your nose and notice the contact points of your spine. **Does your low back feel flatter? Heavier? Softer? More space?**

This transition serves two purposes: it calms the nervous system and lets your body reorganize before the next release.

Now breathe and listen. What needs releasing next? Or is it rest time?

B. THE BOTTOM POSITION: ILIOPSOAS TENDON INSERTION

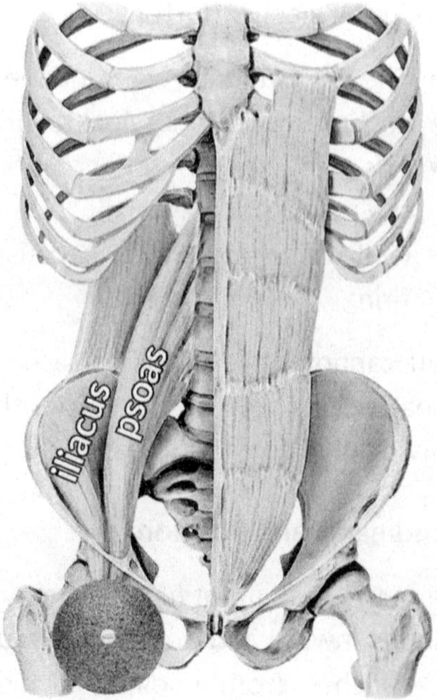

This is where the iliopsoas *(psoas and iliacus)* tendons join before inserting into the lesser trochanter *(leg)*. It's often the tightest restriction point and critical for full hip release.

Location: Approximately 2–3 inches below the pubic bone, along the inner thigh near the bone *(not directly on it)*.

Technique:

- Lie face down or on your belly
- Place the **purple** ball at the landmark, close to the bone but not pressing directly on it
- Gently externally rotate the leg slightly to open access to the tendon

Activate the breath engine: 3-5 pranayama breaths to establish the pattern. Direct each exhale into the tendon: The pressure should feel deep and focused, often referring into the groin or hip crease.

Count every breath to maintain focus
Stay 5–10 minutes per side.

This position bridges the psoas and iliacus work, once you release this combined tendon insertion, the entire front-body pattern begins to let go.

C. DETAILED BALL POSITIONING FOR ILIACUS RELEASE

The psoas drives spinal compression. The iliacus drives hip dysfunction. The iliacus lines the inside of the pelvic bowl from the iliac crest to the lesser trochanter, where it joins the psoas tendon. While the psoas pulls on the lumbar spine, the iliacus pulls directly on the femur, tilting the pelvis forward, rotating the hip internally, and compressing the sciatic nerve along the pelvic floor as it exits through the pelvic outlet.

When the iliacus shortens:

- The pelvis tilts forward independent of spinal position
- Hip internal rotation locks, limiting gait and stride
- The sciatic nerve gets compressed between muscle and bone along the pelvic sidewall
- Glute activation fails because the hip geometry prevents proper firing

You cannot achieve full release without addressing both muscles. The psoas decompresses the spine; the iliacus frees the hip and opens the pelvic outlet for the nerve.

Landmarks and Position:

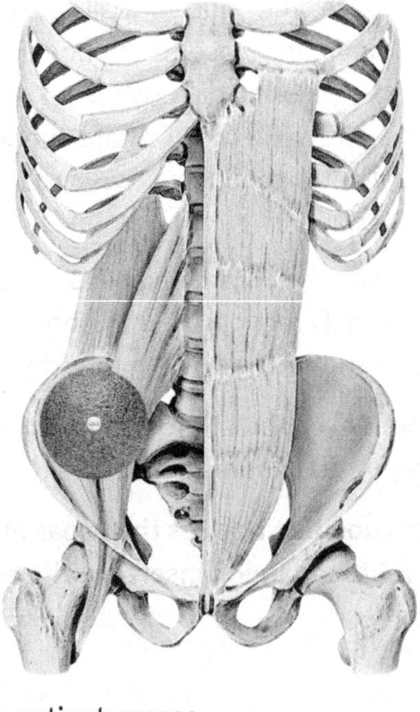

From the ASIS *(front hip bone)* move slightly inward and posterior, about 3–4 inches from midline at hip-bone level, just inside the ridge of the pelvic bowl.

<u>Position 1:</u> Face Down *(Primary)*
Place the **purple** ball on the landmark, elevated on 1–2 books if needed. Lie face down, angled slightly toward the working side so the ball presses into the bowl rather than onto bone. Same-side leg can be straight or slightly bent. Opposite leg extended. Let your weight settle gradually, the iliacus sits deeper than the psoas and requires patient access.

<u>Position 2:</u> Side-Lying *(Alternative)*. Lie on your side with the ball positioned just inside the front rim of the pelvis. Bottom leg straight, top leg bent forward for balance. Angle your torso slightly forward so pressure directs into the bowl, not onto the bony ridge.

Adjusting Pressure:

- **More:** Straighten bottom leg fully, relax abdomen, sink weight
- **Less:** Prop on forearm, bend knees, shift weight back slightly

What You Should Feel

0–2 min: Focused pressure along the inside of the pelvic bowl, often sharper than psoas. Activate the breath engine. Referral into the groin, inner thigh, or hip crease is common, this is the nerve pathway opening.

2–5 min: Surface tension eases, ball settles deeper into the bowl. Continue counting breaths. Direct each exhale into the pelvic bowl.

5–10 min: Deep release; warmth spreading through hip joint, easier hip rotation. The balloon fills and empties, fills and empties, softening the tissue with each cycle.

10–15 min: Full softening; when you stand, the hip swings freely.

The iliacus often feels more lateral and localized than the psoas. You may sense the difference between the two muscles, the psoas as a vertical column near the spine, the iliacus as a fan spreading along the pelvic wall.

Timing: Minimum 10 minutes per side. If one hip rotates forward or feels tighter, spend up to 20 minutes on that side.

Access Variations

If face-down positioning is difficult: Side-lying corridor: Ball just below lower ribs at the pelvic brim, angled toward the spine. Breathe slowly and allow organs to shift as you sink.

D. RELEASING THE CHEST AND SHOULDER - THE DIAGONAL CONNECTION

One-sided sciatica mirrors one-sided upper-body tightness. A forward, collapsed shoulder on one side shortens the anterior fascial line running from pectoralis (chest) through the diaphragm directly to the psoas on the opposite side. This creates a diagonal pull: tight right shoulder rotates the ribcage right, pulling the left psoas forward, tilting the left hip, compressing the left sciatic nerve. Releasing the pectoral fascia evens diaphragmatic pull and unwinds the spiral running from shoulder to opposite hip.

When You Need This Release

Based on the rotation testing you performed in Chapter 5, you already know if you need opposite shoulder release. Approximately 30-40% of people with sciatica need this to fully resolve the diagonal pattern.

If your right hip rotated forward: Release the left pec
If your left hip rotated forward: Release the right pec

Always work the opposite shoulder from the compressed hip.

Technique

Stand facing a wall or door frame. Place the **purple** ball *(faded here so you can see fascial lines)* just inside your shoulder joint where pec major meets the shoulder and then toward the collar bone and sternum, and the wall.

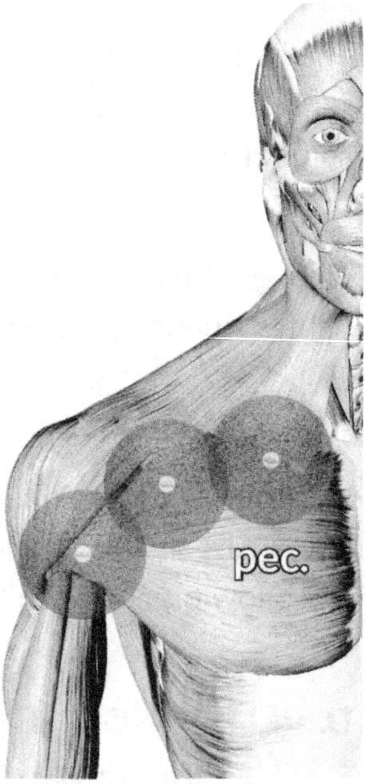

Lean until you feel steady pressure. Micro-shift left or right to locate the densest spot.

- Activate the breath engine: 3-5 pranayama breaths into the chest
- Direct each exhale from the chest
- Let the shoulder drop down and back

Count every breath to maintain focus. Stay 1–3 minutes per position, breathing deeply.

What You Should Feel

Spreading warmth across the front of the chest, rib expansion, and easier breathing. When the pecs soften, the shoulders naturally settle back, the rib cage opens, and the diaphragm moves freely, decreasing tension through the entire anterior chain and pelvis.

Timing: 3–5 minutes, you may only need to release one side, the opposite side of the sciatica.

E. PIRIFORMIS RELEASE - UNLOCKING THE DEEP HIP

The piriformis stabilizes what the psoas destabilized.

When anterior structures pull the pelvis forward, the piriformis contracts to stabilize the sacroiliac joint, and ends up clamping the sciatic nerve that passes directly beneath it (or through it in 20% of people). This is the third and final compression point, if it is needed.

The piriformis runs from the sacrum's lateral edge to the greater trochanter. Releasing it restores balance between front and back of the hip and frees the nerve in the deep hip before it descends the leg.

Locating the Piriformis

Visualize a diagonal line from your sacrum's outer edge to the bony knob on the side of your thigh *(greater trochanter)*. The piriformis lies along that path, deep to the glute maximus *(shaded)*.

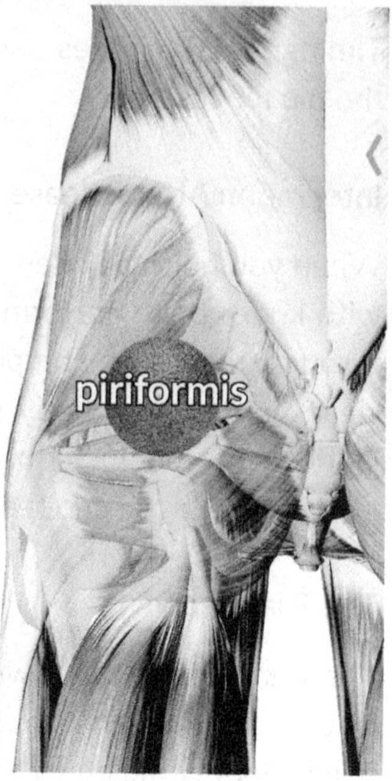

Position 1: Seated or laying on the Floor

- Sit supported or lay with knees bent
- Place the green ball *(or purple for broader pressure)* under one buttock along the sacrum-to-trochanter line
- Cross the same-side ankle over the over the opposite knee, a figure-4 position. This externally rotates the hip and exposes the muscle. Go slow
- Shift your weight slowly an inch at a time until you locate the dense, tender strip, Stop there. Stay still.
- Activate your breath engine: 3-5 breaths. Direct each exhale from the piriformis: Count every breath

Adjusting Pressure:

Increase: Lean more weight onto that side and let the knee drop outward
Decrease: Keep more weight on your hands behind you or uncross the legs

<u>**Position 2:**</u> Side-Lying Alternative *(maybe do this one on your bed or sofa)*

Lie on your side with knees slightly bent. Place the ball under the back portion of your hip near the sacrum. Let the top leg cross forward for balance. Sink slowly until you feel the deep line activate.

What You Should Feel

Deep, centered pressure in the buttock. Possible radiating warmth or ache down the thigh as the nerve decompresses. Gradual melting as the muscle releases. The breath balloon fills and empties, fills and empties, softening the tissue with each exhale.

Timing: 5–10 minutes per side. Stay until the intensity drops by half and the hip moves freely.

Integration After Release

When you finish any deep release, move deliberately. Roll onto your back with knees bent. Perform a few full pranayama breaths, complete inhale through the nose, complete exhale through the mouth, to clean and clear, and let your body settle into the floor for two to three minutes. Notice how your lower back meets the floor, often it feels flatter or more even. Stand, walk, and feel how the hips swing more freely.

The Triad *Secret*

These structures don't work independently. Shortened psoas locks your diaphragm. Locked diaphragm prevents full breathing. Dysfunctional pelvic floor completes the trap. You can't release one without addressing all three. This is why breathing comes before ball work. This is why the ball sinks deeper when you breathe fully. It's one system. Release it as one system.

A Complete Myofascial Release Session

Minimum effective *(15–30 minutes)*:

- Activate the breath engine: 3-5 pranayama breaths
- **A.** Pain side psoas: 15–20 min
- **D.** Opposite shoulder *(if needed based on testing)*: 5 min
- Integration: 3 min

Standard *(35–45 minutes)*:

- Activate the breath engine: 3-5 pranayama breaths
- **A.** Both psoas: 15–20 min each side
- **D.** Opposite shoulder *(if needed)*: 5 min
- Integration: 5 min

Complete *(45–60 minutes)*:

- Activate the breath engine: 3-5 pranayama breaths
- **A.** Both psoas: 15–20 min each
- **B.** Iliopsoas tendon insertion: 5–10 min each side
- **C.** Both iliacus: 10–15 min each
- **D.** Opposite shoulder: 5 min - shoulder and chest may be preformed anytime that you feel tight or pulled forward. Once the psoas lets go it is easier to maintain suppleness with movement and breathing.
- **E.** Piriformis *(if needed)*: 5–10 min each
- Integration: 5 min

Frequency:

- **Weeks 1–2:** 3–4 sessions per week
- **Weeks 3–8:** 3–4 sessions per week
- **After 8 weeks:** 2–3 sessions per week for maintenance

Within the First 30 Minutes

Drink water. Myofascial release moves fluid and metabolic waste; hydration keeps tissue supple. Walk or perform light mobility moves instead of sitting. Sitting immediately shortens the hip flexors you've just released.

Quick Reference – Ball Choice and Timing

A. Psoas
Ball: Purple
Duration: 10–20 min/side
Notes: Elevate on books for depth; pain side first for sciatica

B. Iliopsoas Tendon Insertion
Ball: Purple
Duration: 5–10 min/side
Notes: Below pubic bone at lesser trochanter; bridge between psoas and iliacus

C. Iliacus
Ball: Purple
Duration: 10–15 min/side
Notes: Face-down or side-lying; inside pelvic bowl

D. Chest and Shoulder
Ball: Purple
Duration: 3–5 min/side
Notes: Opposite shoulder from rotated hip; 30-40% need this

E. Piriformis
Ball: Green or Purple
Duration: 5–10 min/side
Notes: After front-body release; seated figure-4 position

Position Progressions for Accessibility

If face-down positioning is difficult, progress through these alternatives: Face-Down → Side-Lying → Seated

Each position offers less intensity but maintains access to the tissue. Start where you can breathe fully and relax completely. As tissue releases over weeks, you may find face-down becomes accessible.

If bed or sofa is needed: Some people need a softer surface initially. This is acceptable in early sessions. Progress to firmer surfaces as tissue softens.

Troubleshooting Guide

Can't find the psoas: Lie on back, press fingers 2–3 in from midline below navel, lift knee; the firm band that engages is the psoas, place the ball there.

Too painful: Use side-lying position, softer surface *(bed or sofa)*, or shorter sets; breathe slowly and direct each exhale into the tissue

No sensation: Re-check landmarks, relax belly completely, add elevation with books

Pain refers to groin/leg: Normal, this is the nerve pathway opening. Continue breathing until it settles

Nausea: Lighten pressure or stop for the day

One side much tighter: Spend longer on that side

Contraindications and Cautions

Do not use abdominal or pelvic ball work if you have:

- **Recent abdominal or pelvic surgery (≤ 6 months)**
- **Pregnancy (first or third trimester)**
- **Abdominal hernia**
- **Severe osteoporosis**
- **Acute disc herniation with neurological loss**
- **Bleeding disorders or anticoagulant use**
- **Abdominal aortic aneurysm**
- **Active infection or fever**

Use extreme caution with: IBS or IBD, endometriosis, kidney disease or stones, recent trauma.

Stop immediately for: Continued sharp pain, progressive weakness, prolonged numbness, *(some brief numbness down the leg is normal at first. Reposition, rest, and resume)*, or loss of bowel/bladder control.

The 24 Hours following Myofascial Release

Expect mild soreness or fatigue as the body reorganizes. This may last for two-three weeks depending on your condition. You may also notice emotional waves, sadness, relief, or even anger, as stored tension clears.

Continue gentle breathing and light movement.

Release Progression – What to Expect

Early Sessions: Finding correct landmarks and learning to breathe through discomfort *(7–8/10 intensity)*. Soreness afterward is normal. The tissue is dense and protective.

Middle Phase: You reach depth faster, intensity moderates *(6–7/10)*. Hip mobility improves, sciatica flares lessen. The nervous system begins to trust the process.

Later Sessions: Tissue feels pliable, pressure tolerated *(5–6/10)*. Back decompresses, breathing deepens, fear of movement decreases. The pattern is changing. Less time can be spent on the ball and more time on movement and nervous system retraining with the breath.

Maintenance: Release happens within minutes. You can sense when the psoas tightens and address it immediately before symptoms return.

When You Will Feel the Difference

- After 1–3 sessions: Freer breathing, less lumbar compression, better hip swing
- After 1–2 weeks: Noticeably fewer sciatic flares, improved posture and sleep
- After 4–6 weeks: 50–80% symptom reduction, greater confidence in movement
- After 3–6 months: Sustained relief with maintenance 2–3×/week

DON'T FORGET ABOUT YOUR FEET

When your feet stop working, collapsed arches, stiff toes, tight plantar fascia, the entire chain compensates. Ankles rotate inward. Knees drift. Hips grip. Pelvis twists. The sciatic nerve pays the price.

The tool, **red Backhealer Ball.** Golf ball size.

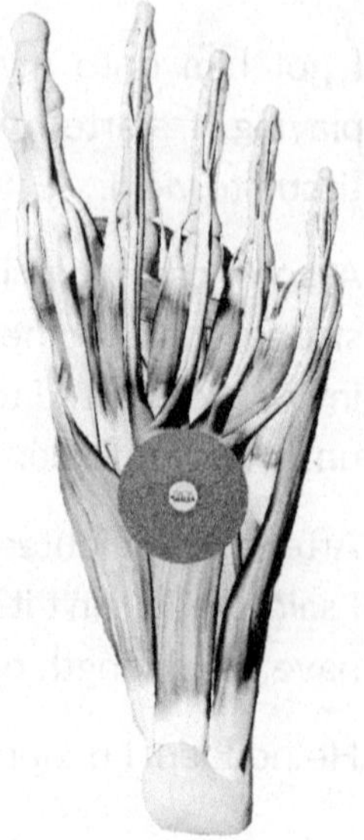

How to Release

- Stand with one hand on a wall for balance
- Place ball **under center of foot**
- Don't roll. Sink. Breathe slowly
- 30–60 seconds center, heel, base of toes, inner arch, outer arch
- 2–5 minutes per foot

Daily or multiple times per day. Never force. Never clench toes.

Releasing the feet:

- Resets mechanoreceptors, which communicate directly with the spinal cord.
- Improves ankle and hip mechanics.
- Reduces pelvic torque.
- Lowers nervous system tone.
- Reorganizes gait.

This myofascial release sequence, psoas, iliacus, chest, and piriformis, and feet is the heart of the Backhealer Method for sciatica. It addresses the true source of nerve compression by restoring length to the front body, opening the three primary entrapment points, and correcting the diagonal pattern that created one-sided symptoms.

You are the director. The ball creates mechanical pressure. Your controlled breath creates hydraulic pressure. Your mind directs where the 13% blood flow increase goes. To the compressed tissue. Clearing waste. Delivering oxygen. Softening fascia. Easing guarding.

When Pain Becomes Emotional Armor

A big guy came in to see me one day. A bodybuilder. Big guy. Bent over for months, could barely walk. His girlfriend brought him in because he couldn't drive himself anymore.

I got him onto my heated table. Room was warm, Frequency playlist playing. I started working on him. Sustained pressure, waiting for the tissue to yield.

A song came on: The Power Is Here Now by Alexia Chellun. This big, strong man, someone who'd built his entire identity around being invincible, started to cry. Deep, shaking sobs. His girlfriend stood nearby, unsure what to do.

After a few minutes, through the tears: "I didn't know I was carrying this." I said, "Wild, isn't it? One minute you're superman. Next minute you don't have the strength of a mouse to stand up straight."

He nodded. I understood.

Everyone Cries

Everyone cries during this work. Not most people. Everyone.

If you've been in chronic pain for months/years, you're carrying years of buildup. Fear. Rage. Grief. Shame. Exhaustion. Disappointment. It's stored in your tissue, shortened psoas, collapsed chest, locked jaw, rigid belly. When the tissue releases, the emotion releases as well.

PAIN AS PROTECTIVE MEMORY

Chronic pain is neurological and emotional, not just physical.

When you first injure your back, your nervous system creates pain as warning: stop, don't move like that, allow healing. That's acute pain, useful, protective, temporary.

Then weeks pass. Months. Years. The original tissue heals, but the pain remains. Your nervous system has learned this area is dangerous. It builds a protective map: this part is vulnerable and must be guarded.

Muscles stay contracted. Fascia thickens. Movement becomes restricted. Your body creates a fortress around the pain site, not because tissue is damaged, but because your brain believes it needs protection.
Emotional armor in physical form.

THE STRESS POSTURES: HOW EMOTION SHAPES YOUR BODY

Your body reacts to emotional stress the same way it reacts to physical threat: it contracts.

When you're afraid, angry, overwhelmed, or grieving, specific muscle groups tighten automatically:

- Fear contracts the psoas — pulls you into fetal position, smaller, protected
- Anger tightens jaw, shoulders, upper back — prepares to fight
- Grief collapses the chest — heart space caves inward, breath shallows
- Shame tucks pelvis, drops head — makes you small, invisible

These aren't metaphors. These are measurable patterns documented in somatic psychology and neuroscience.

When these emotional states become chronic, the muscle contractions become chronic too. The psoas stays short. The shoulders stay raised. The chest stays collapsed.

This is how chronic emotional stress becomes chronic physical pain. You stop noticing. The contraction becomes your baseline. Your body adapts to carrying the weight of your emotional history.

The bodybuilder on my table wasn't just carrying a physical injury. He was carrying years of unprocessed emotion locked in his tissue. He'd spent his life building physical strength as protection. Big muscles, invincibility. But underneath was a frightened man who'd never learned to process fear or vulnerability. His psoas had been locked tight for decades. **When it released, he let go.**

This may happen to you as well.

Maybe not the same way. Maybe not the first session. But at some point you'll encounter the emotional content stored in your tissue:

- Sudden tears with no clear cause
- Waves of grief or sadness
- Anger that feels disproportionate
- Anxiety or fear surfacing unexpectedly
- Old memories
- Shaking, trembling, involuntary movement

This is not a breakdown. This is a breakthrough. Your body is completing a cycle that's been stuck for months/years.

What to Do When Emotion Surfaces

When emotion comes up: allow it. Don't push it away. Don't judge it. Don't try to understand it. Just breathe and let it move.

Protocol:

- Keep breathing: Pranayama, foundation engaged, balloon visualization. Count the breath, in through the nose, and slowly through the mouth. Return to nose inhale and exhale when ready.
- Let emotion move through you: If tears come, cry. If shaking starts, let it shake. If anger surfaces, make noise. Movement completes the cycle.
- Don't make it a story: You don't need to know why. The body is releasing something old. Let it go.
- Stay with sensation, not thought: Notice where you feel it. Throat tightness. Chest heaviness. Belly heat. Stay with physical sensation.
- Give yourself time: When the wave passes, you'll know. Your breath deepens, body softens, spaciousness returns.

Creating a Safe Container

Before each session:

- Dedicate time — 60-90 minutes. Emotional processing takes time.
- Create ritual — Same space, music, scent. Your nervous system learns: this is where it's safe to release.
- Remove distractions — Phone off. Door locked. This is sacred time.
- Set intention — I'm here to release what no longer serves me. I'm safe. I'm ready.
- Five minutes of pranayama — Foundation engaged, 1-2-3-4 inhale, 1-2-3-4-5-6 exhale. Shifts your nervous system into parasympathetic dominance.

Trauma and the Body: When Professional Support May be Needed

Emotional release during myofascial work is normal and healthy. If you have significant trauma history, physical abuse, sexual assault, major accidents, war, childhood neglect, this work can occasionally trigger traumatic memories or dissociative states.

Signs you may need reach out to a trauma-informed therapist or somatic experiencing practitioner:

- Flashbacks or overwhelming intrusive memories
- Dissociation *(disconnection from body or surroundings)*
- Panic attacks that don't resolve with breathing
- Suicidal thoughts or self-harm impulses
- Inability to feel safe

The Gear Shift

You've learned to breathe. You've learned to release tissue. Now you've learned what happens when armor comes off.

Without emotional release, tissue won't fully open. Without tissue fully opening, movement patterns won't stick. Your system has carried a great deal for a long time.

It's ready to get moving!

M1 Foundational Movements.

METHODOLOGY: WHY YOGA POSITIONS

The movements in this book are yoga based. I have practiced these shapes for years. I have taken the shapes from yoga postures and applied specific cues, specific breathing protocols, and specific progressions to make them effective for sciatic nerve decompression and fascial remodeling.

Why I chose these shapes as the foundation:

These are non-moving, isometric holds. When held in correct positions with proper breathing, they remodel fascia better than any other movement system I've encountered. The are safe when used properly.

These shapes are:

- **Accessible.** Many people already know them or have seen them.
- **Equipment-free.** No gym, no machines, no special tools beyond a ball and maybe some props.
- **Transferable.** You can do them anywhere, anytime, hotel room, living room, park.
- **Efficient.** They create length in the front body and strength in the back body simultaneously.
- **Programmable.** Easy to alternate, sequence, and adapt to individual needs.

In the Backhealer Method:

Holds are usually longer: 3-5 minutes minimum, sometimes longer. Fascial reorganization requires sustained pressure. Breathing is continuous and deliberate: Specific pelvic floor engagement that releases tissue and calms the nervous system. Micro-movements are constant: Small adjustments throughout to prevent guarding and keep fascia gliding.

Progression is conservative: You stay at each level (M1, M2, M3) for weeks or months, not days. The focus is therapeutic: These movements decompress the sciatic nerve, restore pelvic balance, and rebuild functional movement patterns. This is yoga adapted for chronic pain recovery. The shapes are familiar. The application is specific.

WHAT M1 IS

M1 movements floor-based, gentle, and completely unloaded. They teach your nervous system that opening is safe without triggering protective responses. These are not stretches, they are openings. You're not forcing tissue to lengthen. You're creating space through sustained holds, controlled balloon breathing, and patient positioning. *Secret.*

Why Everyone Starts Here

Everyone starts at M1 regardless of fitness level, flexibility, or past yoga experience. **Your nervous system adapts gradually.** Fascia reorganizes slowly. The sciatic nerve calms over time, not overnight. If you skip M1 because it looks "too easy," you may trigger protective responses and flare up.

How Long to Stay in M1

Minimum 3-4 weeks of consistent practice. Some people need 6 weeks. Some need 12. You progress when M1 movements feel easy and pain-free, not before. Take the time you need. You may also return to the movements frequently as they are foundational. I still do many of these movements daily.

How to Use This Chapter

A one page visual summary of the M1 movements is provided. Each movement also gets it's own page with a photo and essential cues. You don't need to do all movements in one session. Choose only movements that feel good for your body today. You will develop favorites that make you feel good. Create your own sequences based on what your body needs. There are sample sequences at the end of this chapter.

MASTER PROTOCOLS

Breathing Protocol for All Movements

Continuous nasal breathing throughout. When you feel the need to clean or clear your body then a slow prolonged exhale works nicely.

Summary of the Breath Mechanics - Your breath engine.

- Light pelvic floor and transverse abdominis **engagement** toward your feet, not clenching, just gentle activation like drawing your belly button toward your spine without actually moving
- **Inhale** through nose: ribs lift, belly expands
- **Exhale** through nose or mouth: long, unforced, complete
- **Direct each breath** into the tissue under pressure, balloon breath into the area you want to open.

If your breath becomes shallow, strained, stops, or the mouth opens You've gone too far. Back off immediately.

Intensity: 5-6 out of 10. Enough to feel it working. Never sharp pain.

This breathing protocol applies to every movement unless specifically noted otherwise.

Micro-Movements

Small, continuous adjustments throughout the hold. Tiny shifts. Gentle rotations. Slow circles. Barely visible to someone watching, but profound for your fascia.

MIcro-Movement Examples:

- Toe and finger wiggles
- Light ankle circles
- Tiny rib lifts with inhale
- Small pelvic tilts
- Gentle shoulder adjustments

Micro-movements keep tissue hydrated, distribute tension, and tell your nervous system: **"We're safe. We're exploring.**

Choosing Movements for Your Body

A movement is **right for you** when:

- You can perform it WITHOUT significant pain
- Your breath remains calm and steady
- Symptoms either lessen or remain unchanged when you finish

A movement is **NOT right for you RIGHT NOW** when:

- Pain increases during the movement and continues after you stop
- You rest for ten seconds and pain still builds or radiates
- Your breath shortens, you tense up, or your body feels unsafe

If pain rises and does not calm within 30 seconds of rest, skip that movement for now. Revisit it later after more release work. When in doubt, return to savasana *(dead body's pose)*

Safety Guidelines

- Stop immediately if you experience:
- Sharp, electric, or shooting pain
- Nausea
- Inability to breathe fully
- Progressive weakness, numbness, or loss of bowel/bladder control

Always Do Ball Work First

Opening movements come after release work, not before. If you try to open tissue that's still locked down, you may trigger protective responses.

Minimum preparation:

- Activate your breath engine with 3 minutes balloon breathing
- 5 minutes psoas release *(pain side first for sciatica)*
- Optional: 5 minutes piriformis if tight

As your fascia releases over time, you'll need less ball work. In the beginning though: ball work first, always. This prepares mind and body for movement.

Other Protocols:

- Warm environment (warm fascia opens, cold fascia guards)
- Wait after eating at least 40 minutes
- Use props freely (blocks, bolsters, pillows, straps, blankets, walls)

Hold Times

Fascial reorganization begins after roughly 2 minutes of sustained hold.

Minimum: 2 minutes
Optimal: 3-5 minutes per movement

This is not "do ten reps and move on." This is slow, sustained, patient work.

Elongation Intention

Every movement expresses length from crown to feet. **Never compress into joints.**

Key cue for every movement:

- Reach tailbone toward feet
- Gently flex pelvis floor and transverse abdominis (abs gently pull inward toward belly button.

This maintains elongation, prevents compression, and keeps the lumbar region safe.

Go sloooooow and have fun.

M1 MOVEMENTS - SUMMARY

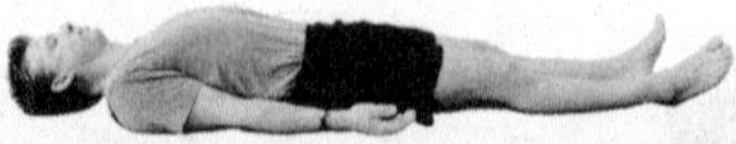

Savasana

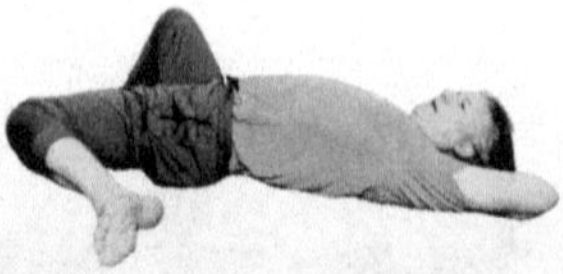

Laying Hip-Flexor

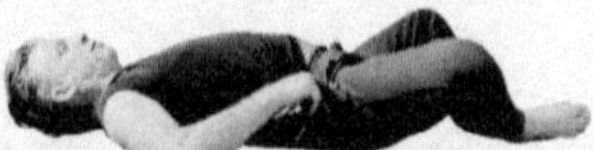

Butterfly

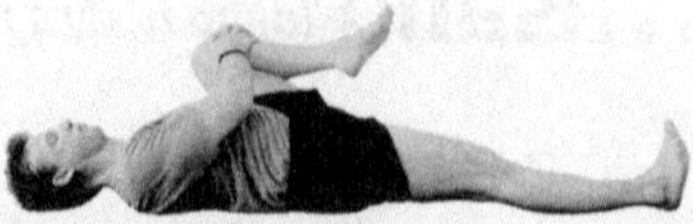

Knee to Chest

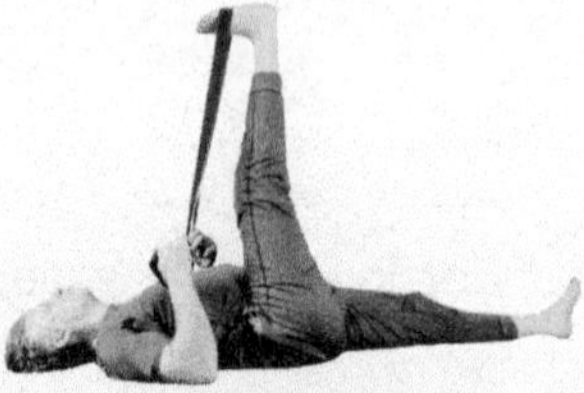

Laying Hamstring

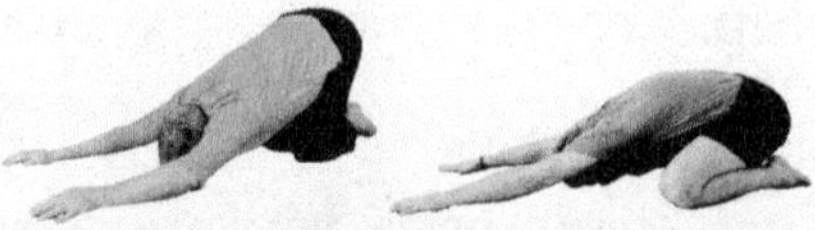

Puppy/Childs

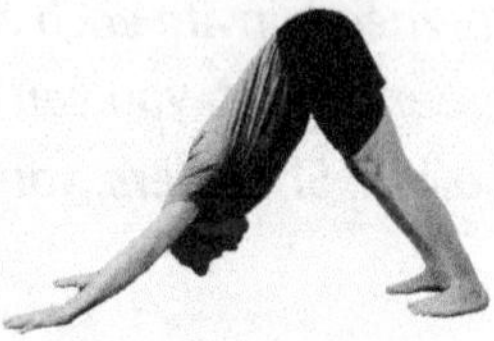

Downward Dog

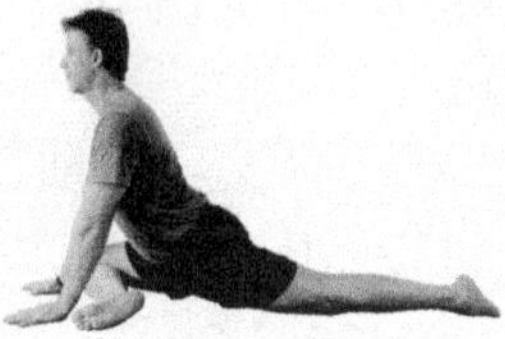

Pigeon

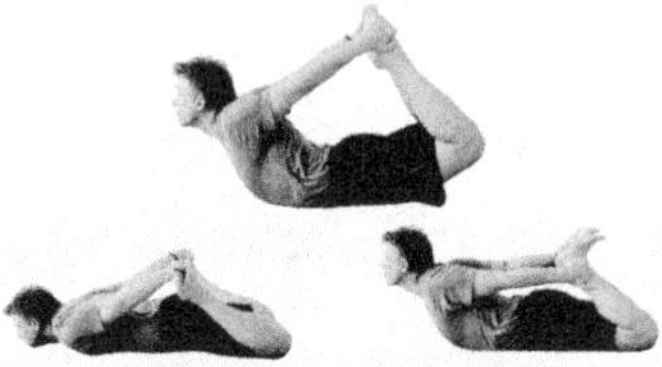

Iliacus to Floor Bow

Lengthen the front
Strengthen the back

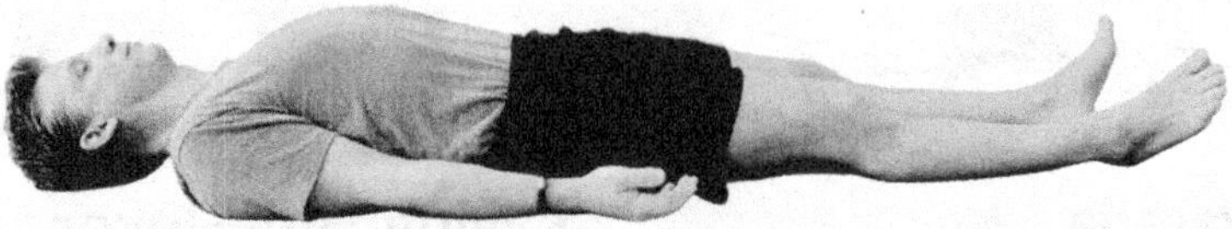

Savasana *(dead body's pose on your back)* M1

Sciatica: This is the safest position for most people, but if lying flat on your back increases leg pain: bend your knees with your feet flat, and/or bolster under your knees, or folded blanket under your pelvis. Keep the bolster/blanket close by for future use.

Setup.

- Lie on your back
- Arms relaxed, palms up
- Feet fall naturally outward, don't hold them together or force them straight
- Head neutral or on small pillow if needed, keep neck long, don't prop chin to chest

Stay.

- 1-3 minutes

Cues.

- Light pelvic floor/lower ab engagement toward feet
- **Activate your breath engine,** full slow breaths
- *Body scan feet→head: invite each region to let go into ground* ***"Feet, you can relax. Jaw, you can soften. Shoulders, you can drop."***

Micro-movements.

- Toe and finger wiggles
- Light ankle circles
- Tiny rib lifts with inhale, settle hips/low back with exhale

Intention: Create a total unloaded and baseline safety state. Begin with this, end with this. Reset here between movements.

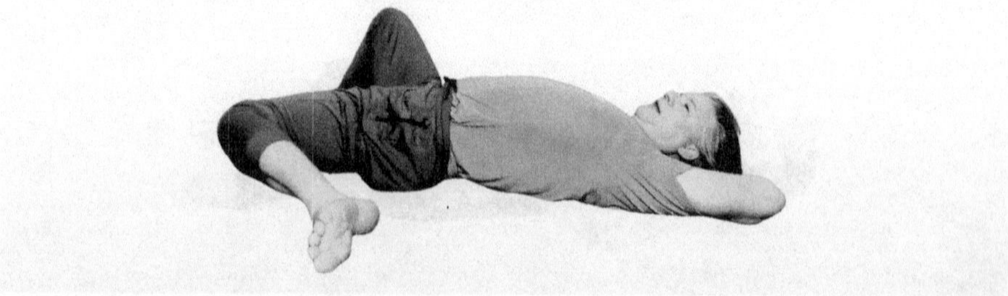

Laying Hip-Flexor **M1**

Sciatica: One of safest long-duration front openers. If groin feels too stretched, slide foot further from pelvis and use prop under knee. If any knee pain, adjust angle or use prop for support.

Setup.

- Lie on your back
- Gently bend one knee and rotate that foot away from midline down toward floor. Knee, foot, and hip form roughly 60-degree angle
- Don't pull foot too close to body, let it rest where it naturally wants to be
- Keep low back on ground via gentle ab engagement
- Opposite leg can be bent with foot flat, or long, whatever feels better

Stay.

- 2-3 minutes

Cues.

- Don't let lower back arch
- Ribs and head reach away from pelvis
- **Activate your breath engine,** full slow breaths
- Tailbone reaches toward feet
- Visualize bent hip joint falling away and out of socket, just a bit
- Let knee and foot relax

Micro-movements.

- Tiny ankle movements on bent leg—point, flex, circle
- Small femur internal/external rotations, let bent leg rotate slightly in/out from hip *(just a few degrees)*

Intention: Releases all hip-flexors, including TFL *(tensor fasciae latae).* Opens entire front body. Passive position, excellent for long holds.

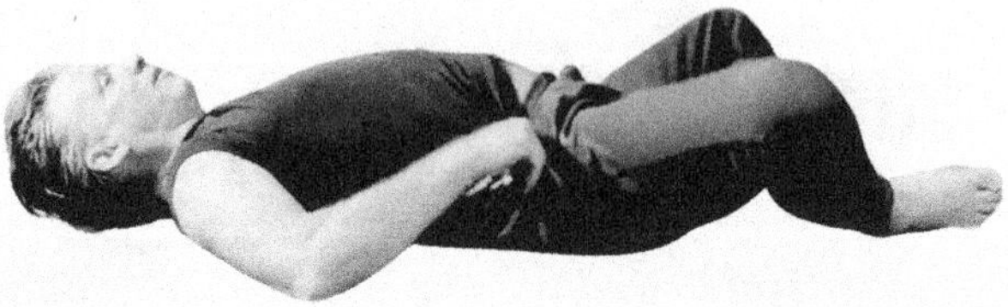

Butterfly

M1

Sciatica: One of the safest front-body openers. If groin feels too stretched, slide feet further away and use props under knees. I do this one id bed

Setup.

- Lie on your back
- Bring soles of feet together
- Knees fall out to sides
- Too much stretch? Slide feet further away from pelvis
- Use pillows or blocks under knees for support if needed

Stay.

- 2-3 minutes

Cues.

- Keep low back on ground via gentle ab engagement
- Both sides of pelvis on ground, don't let it shift or twist
- **Activate your breath engine,** full slow breaths
- Lengthen back of head away from pelvis
- Shoulders on ground

Micro-movements.

- Gentle butterfly flutters with the knees, small openings/closing motions
- Light ankle circles
- Chin nods to lengthen back

Intention: Open adductors *(inner thighs)* and lower psoas/iliacus tendon insertion while entire spine rests on ground.

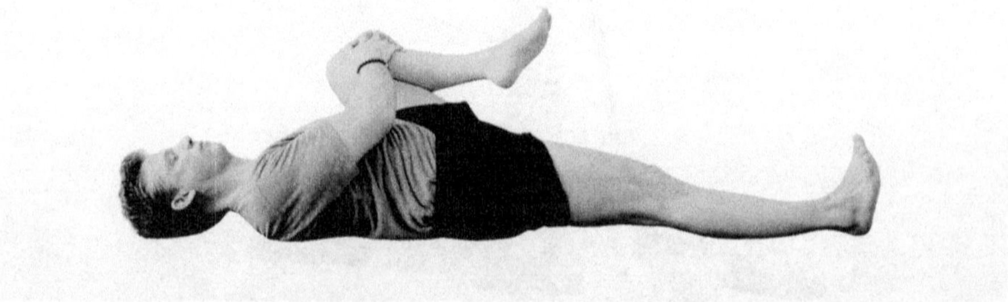

Knee-to-Chest M1

Sciatica: This is for hip decompression, not yanking. Keep the elongation. Don't crunch lumbar spine. If pinching in front of hip, back off slightly, less depth, more breath.

Setup.

- Lie on your back
- Use lower abdomen, not hip flexors, to raise one knee toward chest
- Bring knee just outside rib cage on same side
- Opposite leg stays long and active, reach that leg away from tailbone with flexed foot
- Hold bent knee from behind with both hands, gently pull from your back, feel shoulder blades glide together

Stay.

- 2-3 minutes

Cues.

- Keep low back grounded via gentle ab engagement, don't let lower back arch
- Shoulders stay on ground
- **Activate your breath engine,** full slow breaths
- Back of head lengthens away from pelvis
- Let bent hip joint minutely drop down and out of socket, don't force it

Micro-movements.

- Tiny hip circles, let bent knee make small circles in socket *(clockwise, then counterclockwise)*
- Point, flex, circle foot on long leg.
- Light hand grip pulsing to cue scapular engagement.

Intention: Decompress hip joint. Lengthens groin and hip flexors. Creates opposing forces in pelvis.

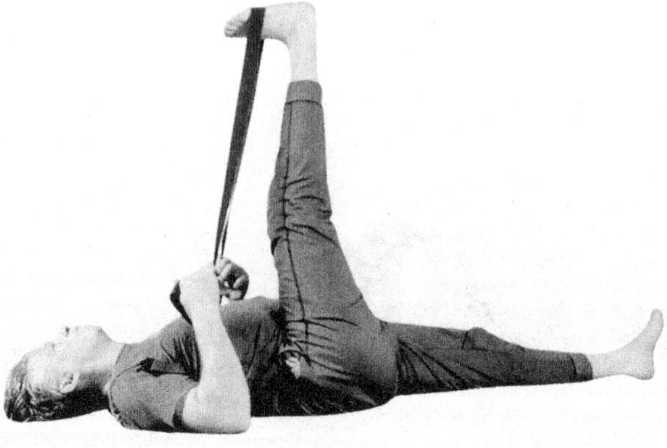

Laying Hamstring M1

Sciatica: If this lights up sciatic tension, unlock knee slightly and emphasize breath over depth. Goal is length in back of leg without irritating nerve. If "zinging" or electrical sensations, back off, you're pulling on nerve, not fascia.

Setup.

- Lie on your back
- Raise one leg using lower abdomen, keep pelvis stable
- Loop Backhealer yoga strap around ball of foot
- Hold band with both hands
- Pull shoulder blades down toward hips, don't shrug shoulders up
- Spine flat on ground, both sides of lower back touching mat
- Opposite leg stays active and long, flex that foot and reach it away from tailbone

Stay.

- 2-3 minutes

Cues.

- 50% pull from hands, 50% push with breath, don't yank leg toward you
- Lock out back of knee on raised leg, straighten completely *(or unlock slightly if creates sharp pain or intense sciatic tension)*
- **Activate your breath engine,** full slow breaths
- Keep spine flat on ground
- Feel hip joint of raised leg falling down into ground as heel presses toward ceiling

Micro-movements.

- Point and flex foot on raised leg
- Micro external/internal hip rotations, let raised leg rotate slightly in/out from hip socket *(just a few degrees)*

Intention: Opens hamstrings and calves. Reorganizes spinal curvature. Creates separation in both side of your pelvis.

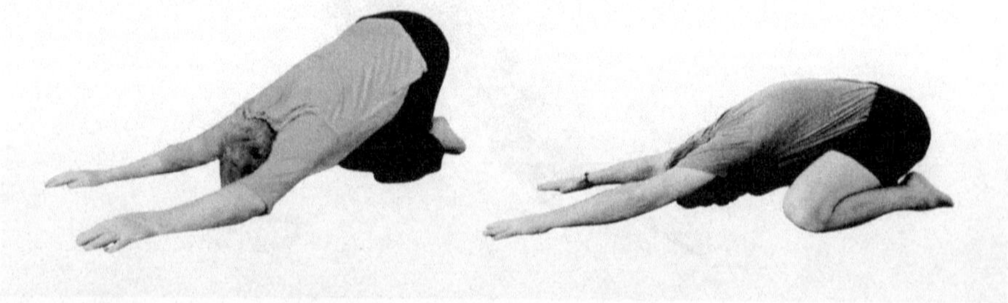

Puppy/Childs M1

Sciatica: Excellent for reducing lumbar tone and decompressing lower spine. Most people with sciatica love this progression. If knees are sensitive, fold blanket under them or use Knee-to-Chest instead.

Setup.

- Start on hands and knees
- Walk knees wide, out toward edges of mat
- Arms juust outside shoulder-width, hands fully pressurized, spread fingers and press through palms

Micro-movements.

- Puppy: Tiny sit bone lifts toward ceiling. Fingertip "crawl" forward on exhales.
- Child's: Slow pelvic rocks. Side-to-side hip shifts.

Stay.

- 1-2 min Puppy, 2-3 min Child's

Cues.

- Puppy phase: Push sit bones HIGH toward ceiling, keep hips elevated, don't sit back yet
- **Activate your breath engine,** full slow breaths
- Belly button pulls inward and chest/forehead relax to ground, arms stay long
- Natural transition: When mid-back and shoulders soften *(1-2 min)*, your body will want to fold deeper
- Child's phase: NOW let bum drop back toward heels, hips fold completely
- Relax front hips fully, let them soften into ground
- Point toes back, don't curl them under

Intention: Create a total unloaded and baseline safety state. Begin with this, end with this. Reset here between movements.

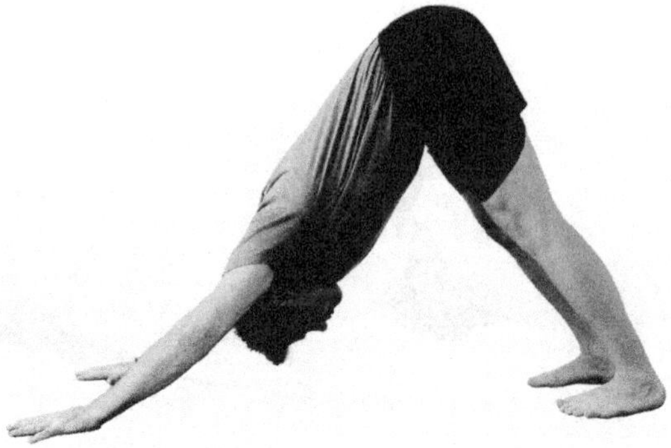

Downward Dog M1

Sciatica: Critical for restoring proper pelvic tilt. Tight hamstrings pull pelvis into posterior tilt, reducing lumbar lordosis and compressing sciatic nerve. If pain increases, bend knees more, raise heels, lengthen spine first. Prioritize pelvic lift over heel drop.

Setup.

- Start on hands and knees
- Tuck toes under. Use lower abs to push sit bones toward sky, belly button lifting pelvis
- Let heels draw down toward ground, don't have to touch, just move in that direction
- Straighten legs as much as you can while keeping spine long
- Hands shoulder-width, fingers spread wide, gripping ground. Press firmly through palms and fingertips
- Push chest through arms toward feet
- Let head hang heavy

Cues.

- Sit bones to ceiling. Heels to ground
- Create space in chest and shoulders as you open chest toward feet
- **Activate your breath engine,** full slow breaths
- Feel abs lifting pelvis, core-driven, not just arm-driven
- Breathe up into pelvis and down through back into head

Micro-movements.

- Pedal feet, alternately bending one knee while other leg straightens
- Small scapular protraction/retraction

Stay.

- 30 seconds -3 minutes

Intention: Release back of legs so pelvis can maintain healthy tilt. Full posterior chain opening.

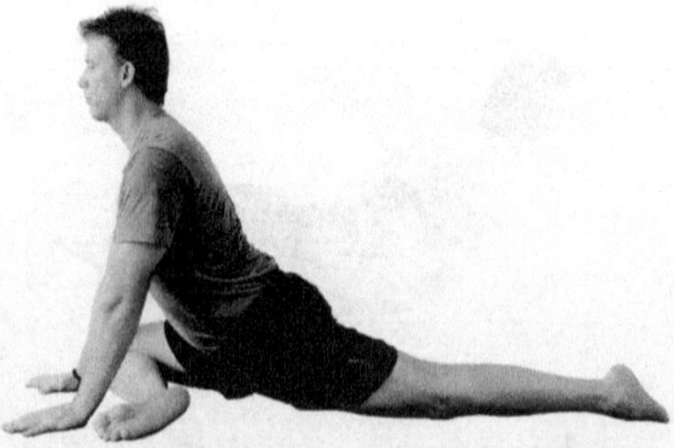

Pigeon M1

Sciatica: Particularly powerful for piriformis-related sciatica once the front body is open. If pain increases, the front body still needs releasing. Try knee to chest.

Setup.

- Bring right knee forward, place behind right wrist. Right foot slides across toward left hip
- front shin can be perpendicular *(more advanced)* or angled back toward hip *(easier)*, start easier
- Extend left leg straight back, top of foot on ground. Keep hips square
- Let front hip relax toward ground

Cues.

- Lift from low abs as tailbone reaches toward back heel
- **Activate your breath engine,** full slow breaths
- **Use arms for support until front hip stops holding you up and starts releasing**
- **This is surrender, let hips rest and open, don't fight gravity**

Stay.

- 2-5 minutes

Micro-movements.

- Use micro-movements in early phase only, tiny pelvis squares, gentle rear-leg tibia rolls, breath-led chest lifts.
- Once front hip is settling, reduce micro-movements.

Intention: Flex one side of pelvis forward while other extends back. Open glutes, rotators, and hip flexors.

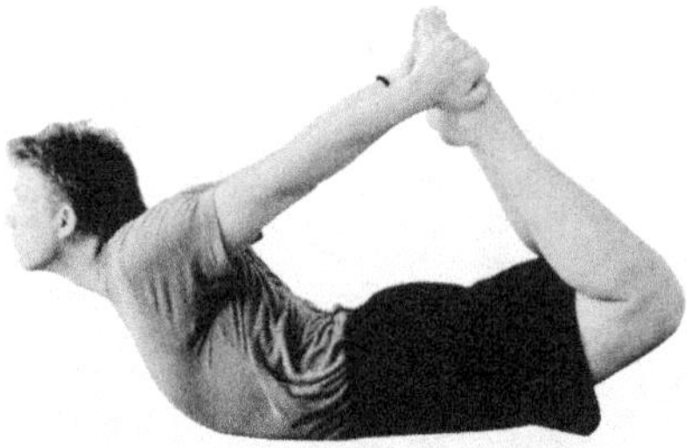

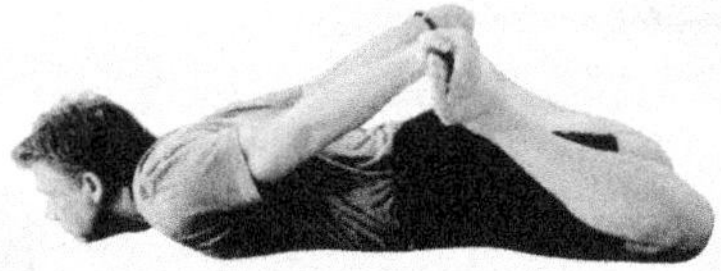

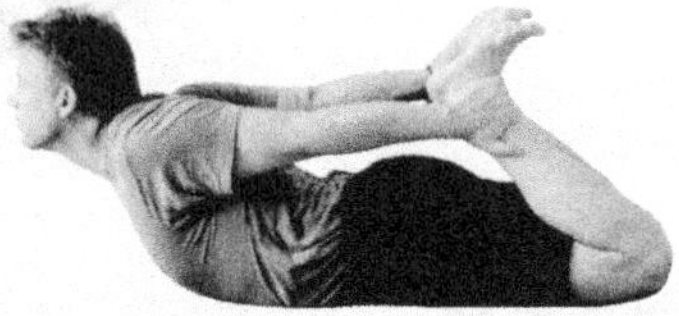

Iliacus Opener to Floor Bow M1

Sciatica: Safest front hip decompressor without lumbar shear. ONLY progress to Floor Bow when Iliacus feels completely comfortable. No lumbar pinching.

Setup.

- Lie on stomach
- Bend knees and reach back for **inside of one foot** with same-side hand, then other foot with other hand. If too difficult: Start with just one leg, reach back for one foot only. If can't reach comfortably, use the Backhealer yoga strap around each foot
- Chin or forehead rests on ground

Micro-movements.

- **Iliacus:** Small ankle turns.
- **Floor Bow prep:** Micro knee presses downward. Tiny chest lifts synced to breath.
- **Floor Bow full:** Minimal micro-movements. Mostly breath-led micro-pulses.

Intention:
Unloaded front-body opening.

Cues.

- **Iliacus:** Pull each foot away from midline toward ground, out and down
- Upper body relaxed, forehead/chin on ground
- Let hips and glutes relax
- **Floor Bow prep.** When ready, shift grip to outside and grab ankles
- Knees press down toward ground and inward. Feet kick away from tailbone
- Lift chest from behind heart using low abs from pubic bone upward
- Opposition between knees pressing down and feet kicking away creates the lift
- **Floor Bow full:** Grab toes with full hand, thumb included
- Let chest round skyward, upper body curves toward sky
- Legs extend out of hips, shoulders roll back and down toward hips
- Build slowly, breath by breath, **don't yank yourself into position**

M2 Movements.

WHAT M2 IS

Congratulations, you have already come a long way!

M2 is not a replacement for M1. It's an addition. Keep doing the M1 movements that worked. Add M2 when you're ready, when M1 feels easy and mostly pain-free. M2 movements are partially loaded. You're sitting, kneeling, or on hands and knees. Your core has to hold you in space while you open. This teaches you to be open AND upright at the same time. This is more demanding than lying on the floor, but it's also more functional.

Most people aren't ready for M2 until 3-4 weeks into consistent M1 practice. Some need 6-8 weeks. Don't rush this.

What Changes from M1

Four key differences:

Partial Loading
In M1, the floor supported you completely. In M2, you're partially loaded, sitting, kneeling, or in positions where your muscles actively hold you. This is more demanding but more functional.

Longer Holds

M1 holds were 2-3 minutes, sometimes 5. M2 holds are 3-5 minutes, sometimes longer. You're asking your body to do more complex work, release AND stability at the same time. That takes time for the nervous system to organize.

Breath-Led Strength

In M1, breath was the primary tool for release. In M2, breath becomes structural. It's not just releasing, it's also engaging your core to hold the new length you've created. Your transverse abdominis starts to fire. Your pelvic floor coordinates with your diaphragm. Your obliques wake up.

This is where strength develops through alignment, not through force.

Dynamic Entry

In M1, you used micro-movements throughout. In M2, you use micro-movements at the beginning of each movement to find alignment and safety. Once you're positioned and balanced, you reduce micro-movements and let breath become the active element. In strong backward bends or heavily loaded shapes, you stay more still once you've found alignment. **Breath replaces motion as the way you continue to open.**

How Long to Stay with M2

Minimum 4 weeks of consistent practice. Some people need 6-8 weeks. You progress when M2 movements feel like they're building strength and integration, not just surviving them. We always practice the movements that work for us.

Prerequisites

You should be mostly pain-free in M1 movements before starting M2. If M1 still hurts, M2 will hurt more. Don't progress out of impatience, progress when your body is ready. We don't wan to go backwards, except when we backward bend.

M2 Practice Keys

The master protocols from M1 still apply (breathing, safety guidelines, micro-movements, elongation intention). Review Chapter 10 if needed.

Additional M2-Specific Principles:

- **Entry: Micro-Movements.** Use small, exploratory motions at the start of each movement to find alignment and safety. Tiny pelvic tilts. Small hip rotations. Gentle rib lifts. These help your fascia align before you add load.
- **Set Phase:** Once aligned, reduce micro-movement in stronger shapes or backbending movements. Let breath become the active element. Your body settles into stillness, and your breath does the work of continuing to open.

- **Core Begins to Lead:** Light transverse abdominis and pelvic floor tone hold the new fascial length without lumbar compression. This is breath-driven engagement, not forceful clenching.

Elongation Intention

Crown and ribs lift. Tailbone reaches away. **Never crunch into a joint**. Every movement expresses length from head to feet.

Sciatica Safeguarding

If a movement increases symptoms and the increase does not settle within ten seconds of rest, regress the depth or return to M1 for that day. Pain is information, not failure.

M2 MOVEMENTS - SUMMARY

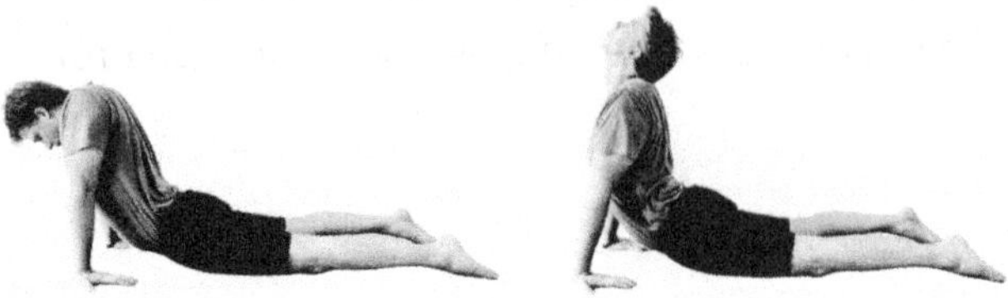

Extended Cobra

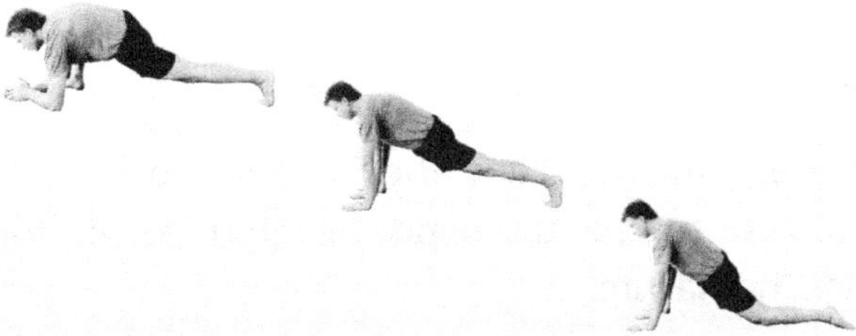

Lizards

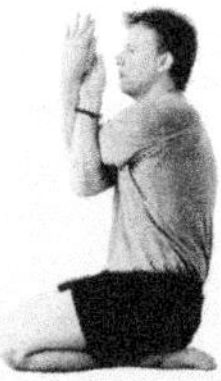

Seated ½ Eagle

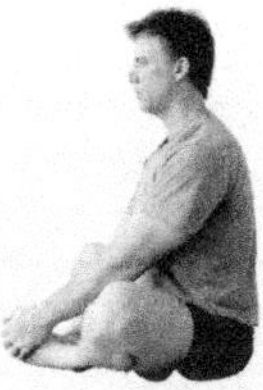

Seated Butterfly

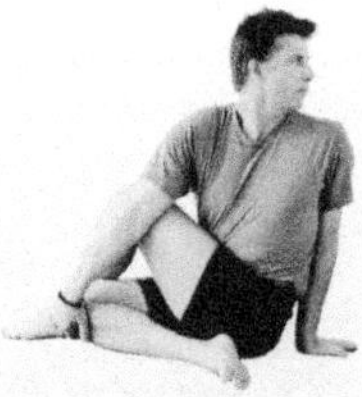

Seated Side Twist

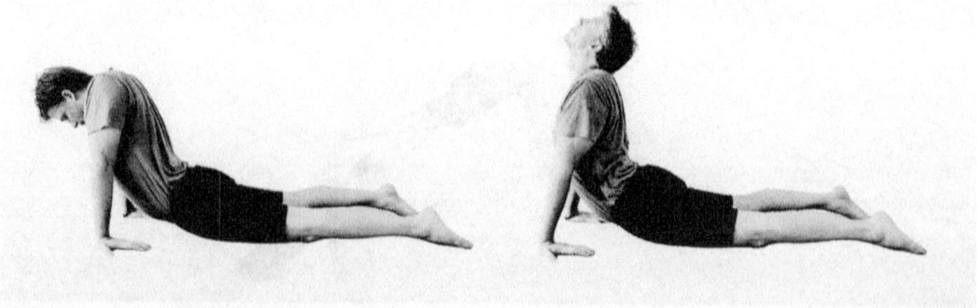

Extended cobra M2

Sciatica: Start with head-down phase, safer and focuses on decompressing back of neck. If lumbar pinching, widen hand placement, bend arms more, and re-engage lower abs. ONLY progress to head-up when head-down feels completely comfortable. If symptoms increase, exit to Puppy/Childs.

Setup.

- Lie on stomach
- Place hands beside chest
- Straighten arms to lift torso, hips/low back/legs
- Don't clench glutes
- Light squeeze between shoulder blades, draw them toward each other and down toward hips
- Lower abs lifts from pubic bone upward

Micro-movements.

- Shoulder blades up and down.
- Tiny chin glides to find sweet spot.
- Head up: Minute chest lifts on inhale.

Cues.

- **Head-down phase** *(neck decompression)*: Tuck chin to chest, look down at ground between hands
- Create space between each vertebra
- **Progression to head-up** *(chest opening)*: When ready, lift chin away from chest. Look upward
- Focus on front of neck and chest as head lifts
- **Both phases:** Tailbone reaches toward heels. Pelvic floor and transverse abdominis draw diaphragm toward pelvis
- Breathe into upper back and neck
- **Don't hold breath, if breath stops, reduce depth**

Intention: Create space between vertebrae and restore spinal curvature. Head-down focuses on back of neck decompression. Head-up opens front of neck and chest. Supported backbend that begins to load spine in extension.

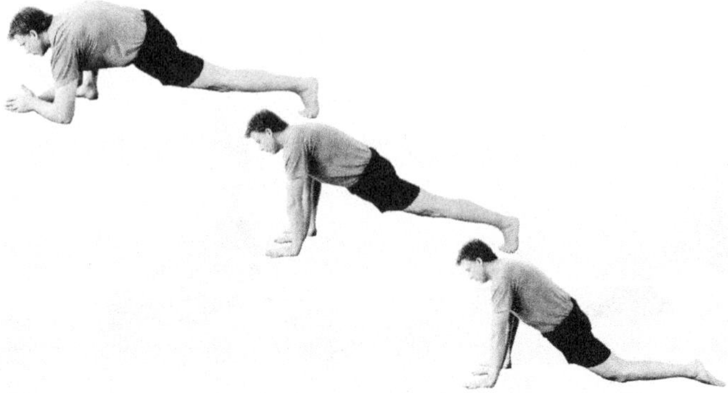

Lizards *(knee down, knee up, knee up elbows down)* M2

Sciatica: Excellent pelvic decompressor. If front groin pinches, shorten stride. Pad rear knee with folded blanket if uncomfortable. ONLY progress to knee-up or elbows-down when first version feels completely comfortable.

Setup.

- Start on hands and knees or downward dog (M1)
- Step foot forward outside hand. Knee roughly above right ankle, don't let knee shoot to far forward
- If hands don't reach ground comfortably, use blocks
- Keep hips square, both hip points facing forward
- Keep back long, neck long, don't collapse chest toward front thigh

Micro-movements.

- All phases: Use micro-movements early, small pelvic squares, gentle rear-ankle movements.

Cues.

- **Knee-down phase:** Knee to ground, shift weight into forward hip
- Feel front hip joint gliding backward
- Feel rear hip gliding forward
- **Knee-up progression *(more strength)*:** When ready, Knee off ground, tuck toes
- Rear leg now straight and active
- **Elbows-down progression *(more depth)*:** Lower elbows to ground inside front foot.
- If elbows don't reach ground, place blocks under forearms
- **All phases:** Lift upper body away from belly button using low abs
- Keep spine long, don't collapse chest onto front leg

Intention: Square hips. One hip extends forward and other extends back.

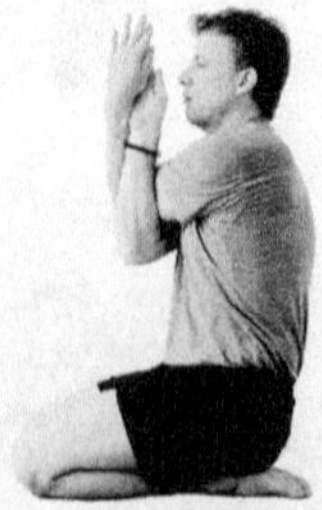

Seated ½ Eagle M2

Sciatica: For thoracic release reducing lumbar overwork. Tight upper back often leads to compensatory lumbar tension. May want to start on your bed or sofa as the fronts of the shins can be tender at first.

Setup.

- Kneel with ankles together under sit bones
- If uncomfortable for knees or feet, sit on block or folded blanket between heels
- Cross right elbow over left elbow
- Bend both arms and bring palms together in prayer position
- If palms don't touch, press backs of hands together
- Lift from belly button using lower abs
- Let tailbone drop toward ground
- Squeeze arms together, press forearms into each other

Cues.

- Let feet point away from body and soften, don't clench feet or ankles
- Feel space opening across upper back between shoulder blades
- Breathe into upper back and neck
- Pelvic floor and transverse abdominis pull diaphragm toward pelvis

Micro-movements.

- Gentle arm squeeze pulses, tiny increases in pressure between forearms.
- Micro chin tucks to lengthen back of neck.
- Tiny rib lifts on inhale to maintain spinal length.

Intention: Can do multiple times a day. Try it standing, sitting, anytime.

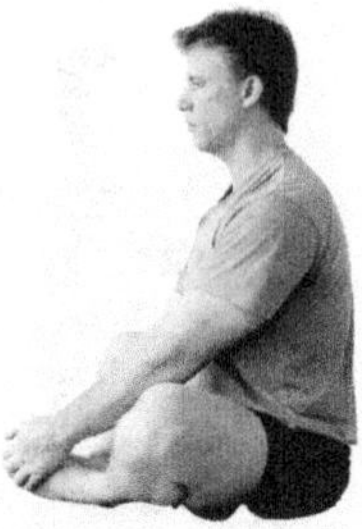

Seated Butterfly M2

Sciatica: If groin feels too stretched, slide heels away from pelvis and prop knees with blocks or blankets.

Setup.

- Sit equally on both sit bones
- Bring soles of feet together in front
- Hold outside edges of feet with full hands, all fingers and thumbs
- Let knees fall out to sides
- Activate lower abs, draw gently into spine
- Lift out of hips
- Lengthen through entire spine
- Let hip flexors relax, use abs
- Don't collapse forward
- Maintain lift

Stay. 3-5 min

Cues.

- Let sit *(sitting)* bones take weight
- Let front hips relax
- Create space through each vertebra as you lift
- Breathe from tailbone upward to top of head
- Each inhale: spine lengthens. Each exhale: hips soften and release toward ground

Micro-movements.

- Gentle butterfly flutters with knees, small opening/closing motions.
- Gentle pelvic rocks, tiny anterior/posterior tilts.
- Tiny shoulder retractions to maintain lift through upper back.

Intention: Ground and release. Open inside of thighs and psoas/iliacus tendon. Strengthen and lengthen core.

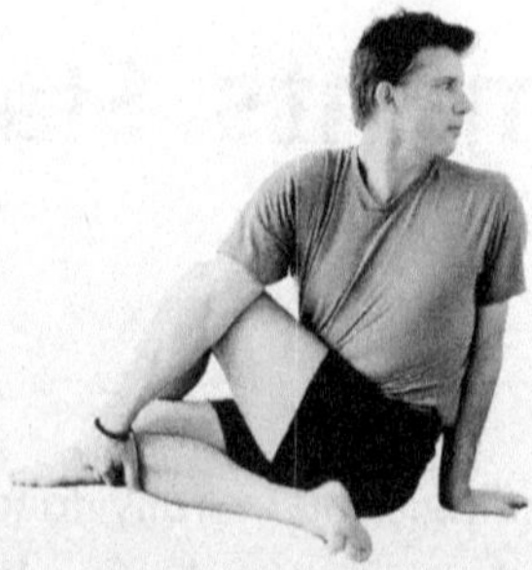

Seated Side Twist **M2**

Sciatica: If rotation provokes symptoms, release hand on thigh instead of hooking elbow over knee and press into knee with elbow. Prioritize lift over twist.

Setup.

- Sit on sit *(sitting)* bones
- Bend right leg under you, foot near left hip
- Cross left leg over so left foot is on ground outside right knee
- Create enough space to keep both sit bones down, this is non-negotiable
- If sit bones lift, adjust legs until both are grounded
- Relax right knee *(underneath)* toward ground
- Lift right arm and hook it over outside of left knee *(crossed over)*
- Left hand on ground behind you at base of spine, fingers turned out
- Lift from lower abs and rotate shoulders and head to left using obliques
- Keep both sit bones down

Cues.

- Hips ground
- Upper body lifts out of hips
- Create space between vertebrae as you rotate
- Eyes track rotation, look in direction you're turning
- Breathe from tailbone up through spine to crown
- Each exhale, rotate tiny bit deeper

Micro-movements.

- Small axial "yes/no" nods with head to keep neck mobile.
- Millimeter-level de-rotation and re-rotation with each breath. **Don't try to twist. Breathe.**

Stay. 3-5 min

Intention: Ground and release. Open inside of thighs and psoas/iliacus tendon. Strengthen and lengthen core.

M3 Movements. Standing

WHAT M3 IS

M3 movements are standing. You're fully loaded, balancing on one or both legs while your body opens and your breath stays calm. This is where breath, release, strength, and movement merge into one coordinated system.

Your core holds you in length without compression. Your feet ground and guide your entire kinetic chain. You can balance on one leg while your body opens. This is functional recovery.

From Front-and-Back to Diagonal Integration

In M1 and M2, most movements worked in the sagittal plane, front and back. You released your psoas, opened your hip flexors, lengthened your front body, strengthened your back body. You addressed the primary compression pattern that causes sciatica: shortened front, overworked back.

Most sciatica doesn't just come from front-back compression. It comes from diagonal tension across your entire body. Right shoulder forward compresses left hip. Left shoulder forward compresses right hip. When one shoulder and chest roll forward, the opposite hip is pulled out of position. The front body shortens diagonally across chest, ribs, and abdomen. The back and hips are forced to tighten just to hold you upright against that diagonal pull.

This creates a spiral tension pattern through your fascia, from one shoulder down across your torso to the opposite hip. When that diagonal line is tight, the sciatic nerve on that side gets compressed.

You can do all the hip work you want, but if you don't address the diagonal pattern, the hip keeps getting pulled back into compression.

M3 movements address this.

Warriors open hips diagonally. Triangle lengthens the entire side-body. Master adds rotation to hip-opening. These movements unwind the shoulder-hip relationship and balance your diagonal lines.

WHAT CHANGES FROM M2

Full Loading

In M2, you were partially loaded, sitting, kneeling. In M3, you're standing on one or both legs. Your entire body weight must be supported while you open. This is the most demanding level.

Balance and Coordination

Many M3 movements require single-leg balance. This rewires proprioception *(body awareness in space)*, critical for people with sciatica who often lose connection to how their body moves through space.

Diagonal and Rotational Patterns

M3 introduces movements that work across the body, opening hips diagonally, rotating the spine, lengthening side-body. This addresses the spiral fascial patterns that feed sciatica.

Stillness Consolidates Strength

Micro-movements happen mostly at entry and exit to find alignment. Once positioned, stillness consolidates strength. Breath does the work of continuing to open.

Feet Ground the System

Your feet become sensory anchors. Ground-to-core integration stabilizes the pelvis and reduces recurrent sciatic flare-ups. Each foot transmits force cleanly up through the kinetic chain when the core functions properly.

HOW LONG TO STAY IN M3

Continue practicing M3 movements 2-3 times per week indefinitely, with M1 and M2 movements practiced as needed.

PREREQUISITES

You should be mostly pain-free in M2 movements before starting M3. Standing on one leg should not trigger fear or significant pain. Your breath should stay calm during challenging M2 movements. Most people aren't ready for M3 until 8-12 weeks into consistent practice.

M3 KEY PRACTICES

The master protocols from M1 *(Chapter 10)* still apply: breathing, safety guidelines, elongation intention.

Additional M3-Specific Principles:

Entry Micro-Movements Only: Use tiny adjustments only at the beginning to find alignment. Small pelvic shifts, chest lifts, or foot adjustments before settling into the movement. Then stillness consolidates strength.

Core and Feet Organize the Chain: Your lower abdomen lifts your spine. Your feet ground and guide knee-hip alignment. This is whole-body integration, not isolated muscle work.

Elongation Intention: Crown and ribs lift. Tailbone reaches away. Never compress into joints. Every movement expresses length from head to feet.

Diagonal Awareness: Feel how movements spiral through your body, from one shoulder across your torso to the opposite hip. Notice how opening one hip affects the opposite shoulder. This is fascial continuity.

Sciatica Safeguarding: If a movement increases symptoms and the increase does not settle within ten seconds of rest, regress the depth or return to M2 for the day. Listen to your body every single session.

Balance of Strength and Ease: M3 movements are challenging, but they shouldn't feel like suffering. If you're gritting your teeth, holding your breath, or feeling panic, back off. Ease is part of strength.

M3 MOVEMENTS - SUMMARY

Warrior 1

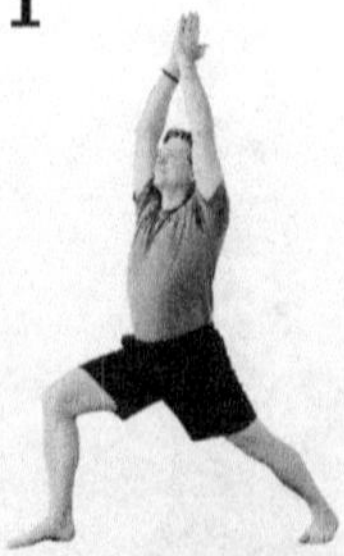

Separate Leg Forehead to Knee

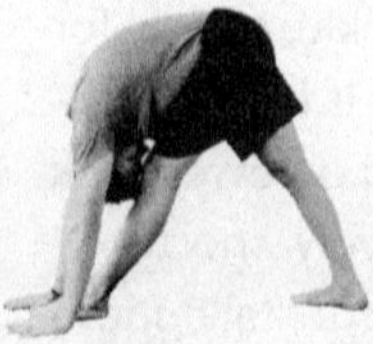

Warrior 2

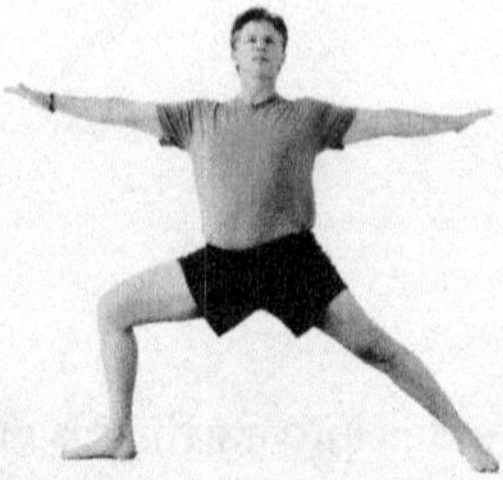

Master

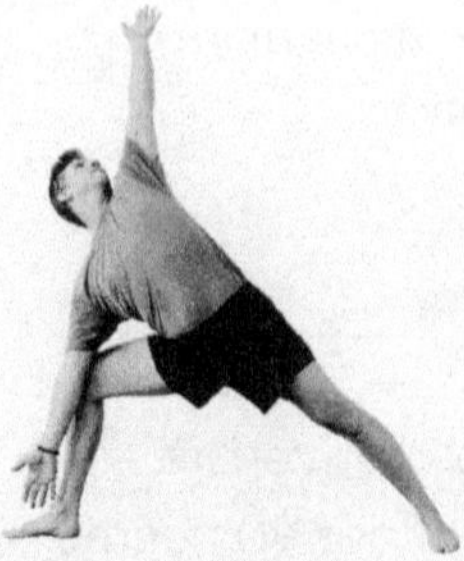

Triangle

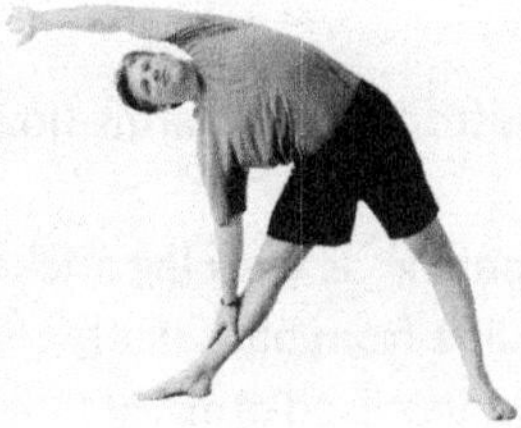

Standing Tree

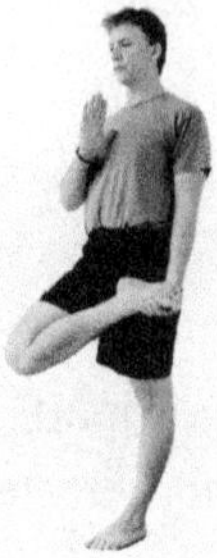

Standing Pigeon

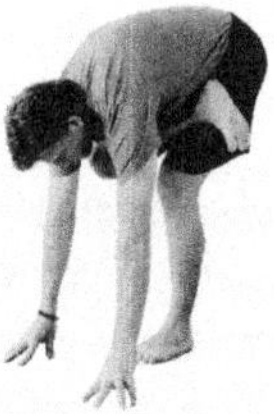

Dancers

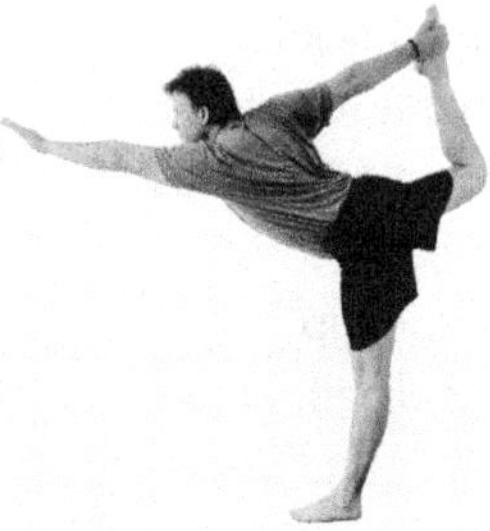

Warrior 1

M3

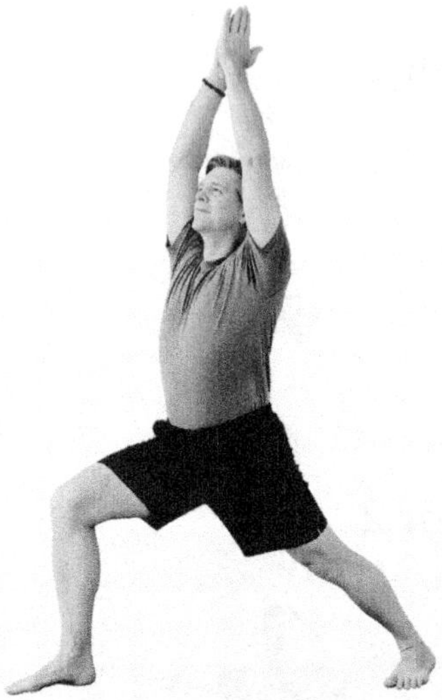

Sciatica: Keep front knee aligned over ankle, critical for pelvic stability. If front hip dumps forward or lower back arches excessively, shorten stance and re-cue: tailbone reaches away, lower abs lift. If back heel won't stay down, turn back foot out more or shorten stance.

Setup.

- Feet hip width apart.
- Right foot out 90 degrees, left foot in 45 degrees
- Bend right knee over ankle, thigh toward parallel
- Square hips forward
- Lift from lower abdomen
- Reach arms overhead from belly, or try reverse prayer behind your back

Intention: Ground back leg while opening front hip and entire front body. Square hips, lift through arms and chest, lengthen psoas and hip flexors. Prepares diagonal hip mechanics.

Cues.

- Back heel presses into earth, this grounds entire movement
- Front knee tracks over second toe, don't let it collapse inward
- Hips square forward, both hip points aim same direction
- Lift from belly button, ribs lift, arms float upward
- Feel front hip opening as back leg anchors
- Notice diagonal line from back heel through front hip to raised arms
- Breathe into front body from pelvis to fingertips

Micro-movements (entry only):

- Small pelvic squares to ensure hips facing forward. Tiny chest lifts with inhale to find length. Gentle back heel presses to anchor. Then stillness.

Separate Leg Forehead to Knee

M3

Sciatica: Prioritize hip-square and abdominal lift. If symptoms increase, shorten stance, keep micro-bend in front knee, lift chest and bend front knee slightly before curling. Don't force depth, let gravity do the work.

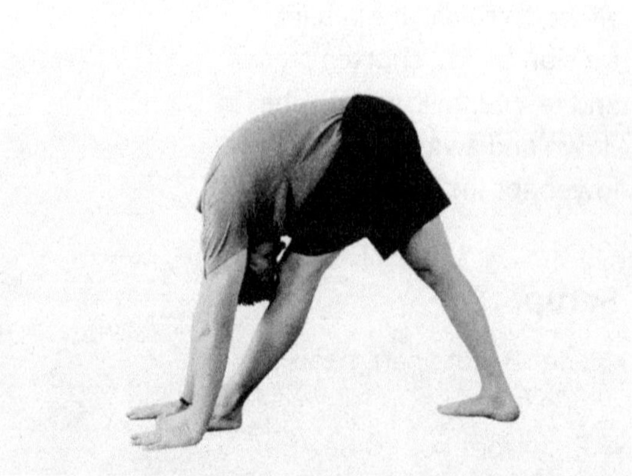

Setup.

- From Warrior 1, straighten front leg. Feet 3 feet apart, back foot turned out 45 degrees
- Both feet flat and pressurized
- Lift arms overhead, use abs
- Slowly curl forehead toward front knee, hands to the knee then the floor
- Round spine deliberately, full spinal flexion, not flat-back fold
- Keep hips square, both hip points facing forward

Cues.

- Ground through lower body as you curl upper body
- Maintain square hips, this is key to entire movement
- Keep both feet flat, if front heel lifts, back off slightly
- Let head and neck be heavy, weight helps lengthen spine
- Feel diagonal release from back hip through opposite shoulder
- Breathe into back from tailbone to crown *(top of head)*

Micro-movements (entry only):

- Tiny pelvic tuck and untuck to find lengthened curl. Then settle into stillness.

Intention: Open entire back body, hamstrings, hips, low back, mid back, upper back, neck. Keep hips square and feet flat. This follows Warrior 1 on the same leg before switching sides.

Warrior 2

M3

Sciatica: Keep front knee aligned, critical. If lumbar tension builds, shorten stance and re-cue: tailbone reaches down and away to the floor, lower abs lift.

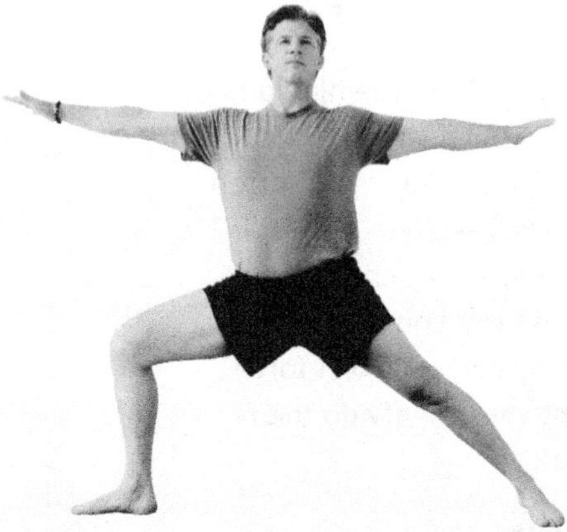

Setup.

- Feet 3 feet apart, heels in one line
- Right foot out 90 degrees, left foot in 15 degrees
- Pressurize all sections of both feet
- Bend right knee over ankle, thigh toward parallel. Push knee back in line with hip, don't let it collapse inward
- Keep hips square
- Lift arms from low abs, shoulder height, parallel to ground. Front arm forward, rear arm back
- Drop shoulder blades down. Look over front hand
- Stay upright, don't lean forward or back

Cues.

- Glutes and hip rotators do hip work, not quads
- Push front knee back in line with hip using outer hip and glute
- Feet pressurize toward each other energetically, engages inner thighs, stabilizes pelvis
- Lift from belly button, upper body light even as lower body works
- Feel diagonal opening from front hip through opposite shoulder
- Notice how opening right hip affects left shoulder, fascial continuity
- Breathe into pelvis from tailbone to crown

Intention: Sit into open, square hips while maintaining easy lift in upper body. Build strength and endurance. Opens opposite hip from Warrior 1, addresses diagonal hip pattern.

Micro-movements (entry only):

- Small front knee track checks, ensure aligned over second toe. Tiny rear foot pressure shifts to square pelvis. Then stillness.

Master M3

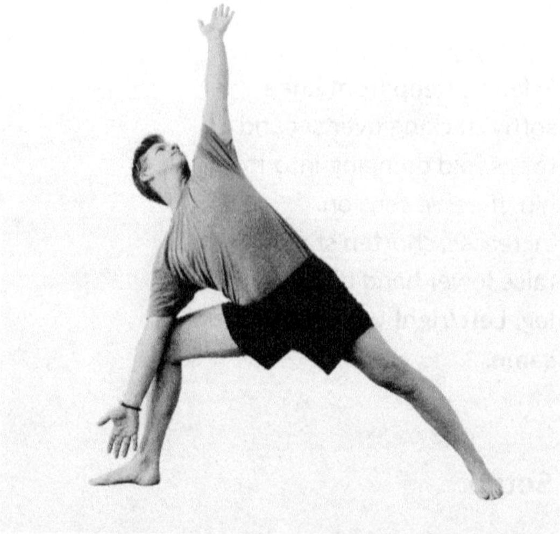

Sciatica: If rotation sparks symptoms, raise bottom elbow higher, rest on knee. Keep spine long, avoid collapsing into front hip.

Setup.

- Start in Warrior 2. Right knee bent, arms extended
- From Warrior 2 depth, rotate upper body to right
- Place left elbow outside right knee. Right arm reaches to sky. Look up at right hand
- KEY: Maintain knee-over-ankle alignment. Don't let knee collapse inward as you rotate
- Maintain pelvic depth. Sit down. Don't stand up straighter just to twist more

Intention: Keep weight in equal in hips while lifting and rotating upper body using abs. Full spinal rotation with side-body length. This is Warrior 2 with twist added, deepest diagonal integration.

Cues.

- Glutes and rotators keep hip stable
- Feet pressurize
- Rotate and lift from belly button, not from forcing upper body
- Feel entire length of spine spiraling
- Notice diagonal spiral from bottom elbow across torso to top hand
- This unwraps shoulder-hip compression on opposite side
- Breathe into pelvis from tailbone to crown

Micro-movements (entry only):

- Micro-moves (entry only): Millimeter de-rotate and re-rotate with breath to find safe depth. Then stillness.

Triangle

M3

Sciatica: Keep front knee softly tracking over second toe. Avoid dumping into front hip. If nerve tension increases, shorten stance and raise lower hand higher on leg. **Left/right will not be the same.**

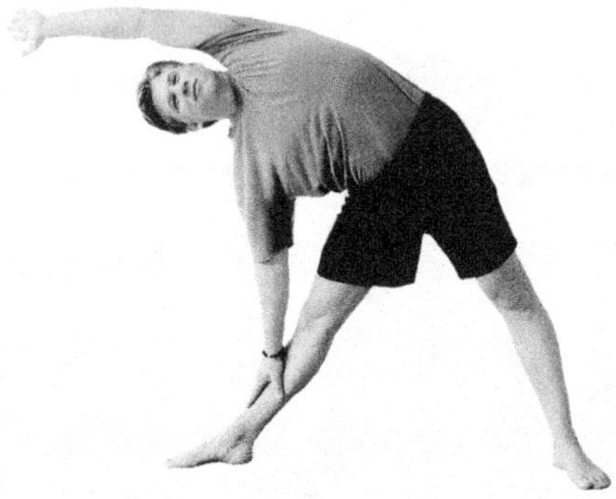

Setup.

- Feet wide, 3 feet apart One foot out 90 degree, other heel lines up in the middle of its arch Pressurize all sections of both feet
- Lift out of hips using lower abs. Hinge sideways to right with long spine, not forward or back, but directly to side.
- Right hand to shin or ankle. **Not on knee.** Keep spine long
- Left hand reaches up
- Stack shoulders
- Head in line with spine Look up to top hand

Intention: Ground lower body while lifting whole side-body out of hips. Spine stays straight, no collapse. Pure diagonal side-body lengthening.

Cues.

- Lift from belly button as legs ground into earth
- Create space in each vertebra as you lengthen toward sky
- Don't collapse into bottom side, keep both sides equally long
- Feel diagonal line from bottom foot through torso to top hand
- This lengthens entire lateral fascial line, key for hip-shoulder balance
- Notice how lengthening right side affects left hip
- Breathe into side-body from tailbone to crown *(top of head)*

Micro-movements (entry only):

- Small pelvis squares to ensure both hips facing forward. Tiny sternum lifts to maintain length. Then stillness.

Standing Tree

M3

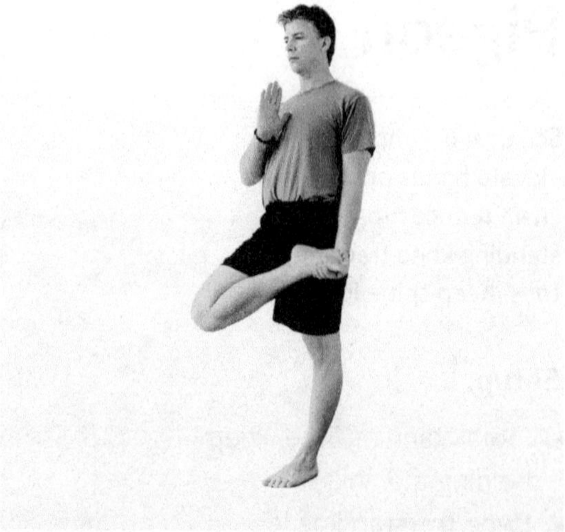

Sciatica: If balancing irritates symptoms, touch wall and reduce knee opening angle. Prioritize abdominal lift over height of lifted leg. Balance work can challenge nervous system. If frustrated or panicked, back off.

Setup.

- Stand with feet together
- Ground through one foot, press through all sections
- Pick up opposite leg, grab ankle. Let knee open to side
- Sole of foot rests against inner right thigh calf, or ankle, never on knee joint.
- If balancing is difficult, keep toes on ground, knee open to side. Eyes 10 feet in-front of you. Or touch wall for support
- Lift from belly button
- Drop shoulder blades down
- Lengthen through back of head
- Fix gaze on one point, drishti it's called. Don't let eyes wander

Intention: Ground and balance on one leg while lifting upper body to sky. Build stillness and focus.

Cues.

- Standing hip is trunk of tree, strong, rooted, stable
- Upper body lifts with ease like branches reaching toward sun
- When you wobble, and you will, return focus to drishti, re-engage core, find center
- Feel vertical lift from standing foot through crown
- Breathe into upper body and neck

Micro-movements (entry only):

- Gentle foot tripod pressure shifts in standing foot, tiny weight adjustments between heel, ball, inner edge, outer edge. Then stillness.

Standing Pigeon

M3

Sciatica: If symptoms rise, elevate hands on blocks or chair, reduce hinge. Keep standing knee tracking over toes. Keep spine long.

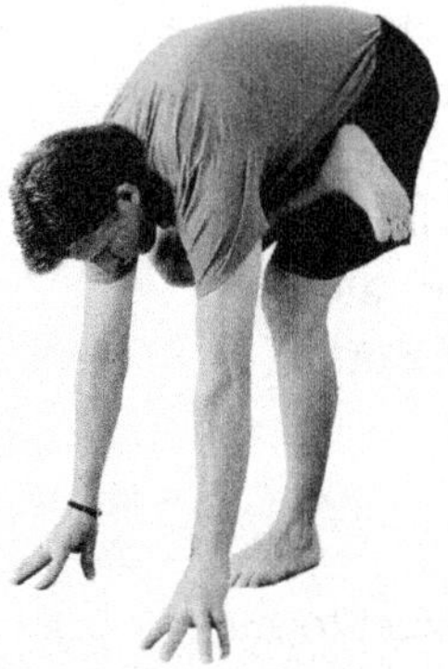

Setup.

- From Standing Tree, keep holding the ankle
- Bend the standing leg slightly
- Hinge forward from hips Hands reach toward ground, use block, ground, or chair
- Foot stays tucked near hip crease
- Push butt backward, bend deeper into standing leg, this opens hip
- Keep spine long, don't round back
- Lengthen from tailbone to crown even as you hinge forward

Intention: Ground standing leg while opening opposite hip. Build hip strength and balance.

Cues.

- Feel left hip releasing and opening
- Engage abs into spine to maintain length
- Let upper body and head relax down without rounding low back
- Standing leg is working, feel glute and hamstring engaging
- Engage abdomen slightly
- Notice how opening left hip creates space in lower back
- Breathe into opening hip and up spine

Micro-movements (entry only):

- Tiny pelvis squares and ankle dorsiflexion/plantar flexion of standing foot to find optimal alignment.

Dancers

M3

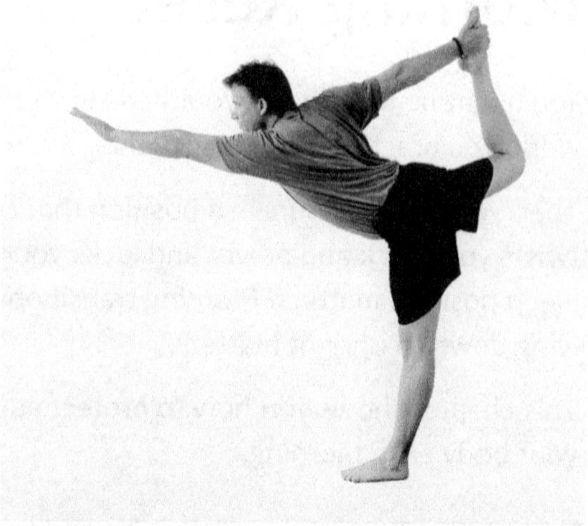

Sciatica: If symptoms rise, keep kick lower, hold wall with free hand, re-cue: tailbone reaches away, lower abs lift. Avoid lumbar hinging, lift from chest, not from cranking lower back.

Setup.

- Ground through one foot evenly
- Bend opposite knee, reach back with same hand to grab foot. Palm wraps around top of foot, thumb included
- Reach arm to sky from belly button
- KEY: Kick leg up and back as you reach opposite arm forward and up
- These opposing forces, kick and reach, create arch and balance
- Keep hips square and level
- Arch upper body out of hips and skyward
- Don't hinge forward, lift up and back
- Fix gaze on one steady point. Drishti

Intention: Balance of strength and ease. Maintain hip-square while hip joint strengthens and opens. Full front-body opening while balancing.

Cues.

- Standing leg is strong, feel glute and hamstring engaging
- Focus on lifting and kicking rather than pitching forward
- This is about grace and ease, not force, if grimacing, back off
- Feel entire front body opening, chest, abdomen, hip flexors
- Notice diagonal line from kicking foot through spine to reaching arm
- Breathe into outstretched arm and chest, fuller lungs help thoracic spine lift

Micro-movements (entry only):

- Small chest lifts on inhale. Tiny pelvis squares to keep hips level. Then stillness and breath.

Sleep, Positioning, and Your Morning Reset

You might be undoing all your healing work while you sleep. You do ball work. You practice your movements. You're diligent during waking hours.

Then you sleep 8 hours in a position that compresses your sciatic nerve, twists your neck and pelvis, and locks your psoas back into shortening. Sleep position matters. Morning transition matters. How you move from lying down to upright matters.

This chapter shows you how to protect your healing overnight and reset your body each morning.

WHAT HAPPENS TO YOUR BODY OVERNIGHT

While you sleep, these processes occur:

Your discs rehydrate. Gravity compresses your spine all day, squeezing fluid out of your discs. At night, pressure comes off and your discs draw fluid back in. By morning, they're fully hydrated and more vulnerable to injury. This is why people throw their back out bending over right after getting up.

Your fascia locks into whatever position you hold. If you sleep with hip flexors shortened, your fascia adapts to that shortened position. By morning, you're starting from restriction.

Your nervous system resets. If you sleep in a neutral position, your nervous system learns: This is safe. If you sleep compressed and twisted, it learns: This is dangerous. Stay guarded.

Your tissues cool and stiffen. Blood flow decreases when you're immobile. Everyone feels stiff in the morning, it's normal physiology. But for sciatica, this stiffness can trigger nerve compression if you don't transition carefully.

Your sleep may be shortening your front body. *Secret.*

YOUR EVENING WIND DOWN

Before bed, if you have time and energy, do gentle unwinding.

Choose one or two movements:

Puppy/Childs
Knee-to-Chest
whatever is needed - you are the Director.

Add breathing: Balloon breathing: slow inhales, long exhales

Set up your sleep position before you're exhausted, arrange pillows, make it inviting.

Sleep environment:

Coolish room
Dark: blackout curtains or eye mask
Quiet: white noise or earplugs
No screens before bed

SLEEP POSITIONS AND YOUR MORNING ROUTINE

Here's the truth: People with chronic pain sleep however they CAN sleep. I've slept on my stomach for 60 years. Is it ideal? No. But it's what works for me.

You might sleep on your side curled up. You might sleep on your back. You might rotate through positions all night. The goal isn't to force yourself into a "perfect" sleep position and suffer through sleepless nights. **The goal is to understand what your sleep position does to your body and adjust your morning routine accordingly.**

The basic structure:

- Preparation in bed
- Transition to standing *(roll to side, push up slowly, stand slowly, check your body)*
- Breathing and hydration *(three balloon breaths, drink water)*
- Standing movements *(specific to your sleep position)*
- Close *(three final breaths, notice how you feel)*

Different movements based on how you slept:

Stomach Sleeping

What happened overnight: Neck rotated 90 degrees, lumbar spine in excessive extension, hip flexors shortened, pelvis tilted forward

Your specific routine:

- In bed: Knee-to-Chest, Puppy Pose
- Standing movements: Gentle neck turns, Warrior 1 *(both sides)*, Standing Pigeon *(both sides)*

Side Sleeping

What happened overnight: Top hip compressed, shoulder bearing weight, the side you slept on got compressed all night

Your specific routine:

- In bed: Knee-to-Chest, Puppy Pose *(focus on the shoulder you slept on)*
- Standing movements: Standing Pigeon *(MORE time on the compressed hip)*, Warrior 1 *(both sides)*

Back Sleeping

What happened overnight: Most neutral position, lumbar curve may have increased

Your specific routine:

- In bed: Knee-to-Chest, Puppy Pose, then Child's Pose
- Standing movements: Warrior 1 *(both sides)*

WANT TO CHANGE YOUR SLEEP POSITION?

Side-lying setup:

- Firm pillow between knees AND ankles
- Small rolled towel at waist if there's a gap
- Body pillow for top arm
- Hips and knees bent at natural angle

Back-lying setup:

- Firm bolster under knees
- Small lumbar support if needed
- Thin neck pillow
- Arms at sides, palms up

Be patient with your body as it adjusts. But if changing position means you don't sleep, stay where you are. Just adapt your morning routine.

YOUR MATTRESS AND PILLOW

Mattress:

Medium-firm is best for most people with sciatica.
Too soft = excessive sinking. Too hard = pressure points. Medium-firm = supports spine while contouring to body.

Replace mattress when you wake up more sore than when you went to bed, or when there are visible sags.

Pillows:

- Side sleepers: thick enough to keep neck aligned
- Back sleepers: thin, fills gap under neck
- Knee support: firm, doesn't compress flat
- Replace regularly

WHAT YOUR MORNING PRACTICE DOES

Every morning, your body asks: How will my back and body feel today?

Your morning routine brings you back to zero. Whatever compression happened overnight, shortened hip flexors, rotated neck, locked fascia, gets released.

You don't start from restriction. You start from baseline.

Through daily resetting, your body learns: I can move safely. I can be free. That's when sciatica loses its grip.

The 90-Day *Secret*

You've learned nine secrets. Here they are:

The Front Body Secret: Your back pain doesn't start in your back. Front body compression, psoas, iliacus, diaphragm, chest, creates the problem.

The Breathing Secret: Pranayama breathing releases the psoas-diaphragm-pelvic floor triad from inside. Ball work releases from outside. Both necessary.

The Diagonal Secret: Sciatica may come from cross-body patterns. Right shoulder compresses left hip. Left chest pulls right hip. Release the diagonals or hip work won't hold.

The Sleep Secret: Eight hours in wrong position re-shortens hip flexors every night. Discs are swollen and vulnerable first hour after waking. Fix sleep position. Protect your morning.

The Opening Secret: Opening isn't stretching. Three to five minutes with breath integration teaches your nervous system the new length is safend permanent.

The MRI Secret: Thirty to forty percent of pain-free people have disc abnormalities. Size of herniation doesn't predict pain. Structure doesn't equal symptoms.

The Triad Secret: Psoas, diaphragm, and pelvic floor work as one system. Can't release one without addressing all three.

The Forces Secret: You can be functional without structural healing. My structure didn't change. The forces acting on it did. That was enough.

The Symptom Secret: Sciatica describes nerve irritation. The cause is usually front-body compression. Fix the compression, quiet the nerve.

Now here's the tenth. 90 Days.

Ninety days is the minimum for fascia to remodel and neurological pathways to reinforce.

After thirty days, habit forms. After sixty days, neural pathways strengthen. After ninety days, fascial adaptation begins.

Less than ninety days equals incomplete change. This is what separates people who read this book from people who use this book and feel better.

What Ninety Days Does

- Day 30: Nervous system recognizes the pattern. Alarm response quiets. Mornings are easier.
- Day 60: Neural pathways reinforce. The triad coordinates automatically. Movement feels more natural. Pain spikes recover faster.
- Day 90: Fascial remodeling begins. Collagen fibers reorganize. Hip flexors hold their length between sessions. The pattern sticks.
- Three months minimum for your body to accept the new pattern as permanent.

Two Outcomes - One tracked data for ninety days. One didn't.

Person A: Felt better after week one. Pain dropped from eight to five. Week two, back to six. Week three, back to seven. Stopped. Still in pain.

Person B: Felt better after week one. Pain dropped from eight to five. Week two, back to six. Week three, back to seven. Looked at journal: trending down despite setbacks. Kept going. Week twelve: pain at one, sometimes zero. Functional now. Same knowledge. Different outcome.

The Pattern

Week 1: Excitement.
Week 3: Doubt. "This isn't working."
Week 5: Small breakthrough. Tied shoe without thinking about it.
Week 7: Plateau. Pain stuck at same level for two weeks.
Week 10: Another breakthrough. Slept through the night.
Week 12: Looking at Week 1 data. Pain dropped from eight to two.

This is the pattern. Expect it.

Why Tracking Matters

Your brain says: "Week seven, still at a five. Nothing's working." Your journal says: "Week one: 8/10. Week four: 6/10. Week seven: 5/10." That's 37% reduction. The data shows progress when pain obscures it.

Marcus wanted to quit at week six. His journal showed fifteen-degree improvement in spinal angle. He kept going. Week twelve: fully upright.

Sarah wanted to quit at week eight. Her journal showed pain dropped from 8/10 to 3/10. She kept going. Week twelve: performing professionally again.

Track or lose objectivity.

The Journal

Track in a notebook, spreadsheet, or use the 90-Day Backhealer Journal (designed specifically for this method with daily pages, weekly reflections, monthly assessments - see Resources).

Use it or don't. But track something. Without data, you're guessing.

Where They Are Now

Marcus: Standing straight. Coaches his son's soccer team. Disc herniation still there. Forces changed.

Sarah: Performs six nights a week. Disc bulge still there. Pain is not.

Me: Sixty years old. Missing discs, spondylolisthesis unchanged. Do seven-minute sequence every morning. Functional, active, pain-free most days.

All three tracked ninety days.

Start Tonight

- Decide how you'll track
- Set alarm ten minutes earlier
- Water on nightstand, balls ready
- Set up sleep position

Tomorrow:

- Seven-minute sequence before phone
- Sometime in your day
- Myofascial Release - 15 minutes
- Movements - 15 minutes
- Track it
- Repeat for ninety days

After Ninety Days

Your pain will be lower. Movement will be freer. Sleep will be better. Journal will show the data.
Then you choose: continue what works or go back.
Most people continue. By day ninety, this is just what you do.

The Facts

Born with missing discs. Grade 2 spondylolisthesis. Severely degenerated L4. Scoliosis. Reverse cervical curve. Spent decades developing this method. Structure didn't heal. Discs still gone. Spondylolisthesis still there. But I'm functional. Not luck. Work. Daily. For years. Still do seven minutes every morning at sixty. This is maintenance, not cure. It works if you work it.

You have the tools. The method is clear.

Ninety days starting tomorrow.

You decide. Pain or no Pain.

Resources

Your 90-Day Reset Journal

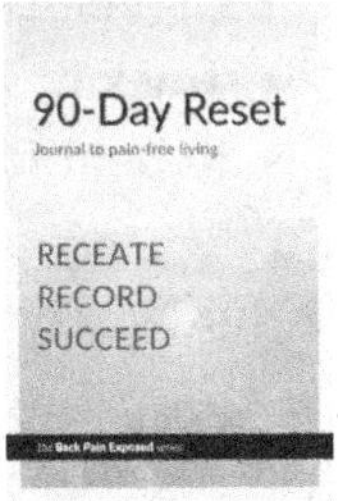

- track your daily practice
- log symptoms
- monitor progress
- **stay accountable through the critical first 90 days**

exlcusively on Amazon

backpainexposed.com - Free companion resources

- Deeper dives into the Science. **Free pdf downloads** expanding on the breathing, myofascial release, and the movements.
- Info on all the books in the series.

Acupressure Ball & Yoga Strap Set

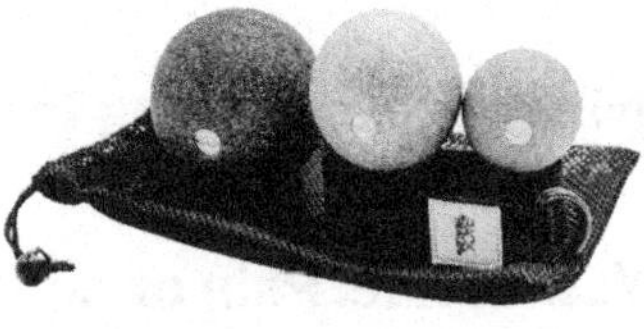

- **Purple** ball *(softball size)*
  - front body releases
- **Green** ball *(baseball size)*
  - glute, hip, and upper back releases
- **Red** ball *(golf ball size)*
  - feet releases and precision work
- High quality yoga strap
- Mesh travel bag

This is the set I use. There are others that may work on Amazon. Pay attention to the sizing.

backspasmrelief.com

Download your **Free** Emergency Back Spasm Protocol with expanded information.

---

backhealer.com

Video demonstrations of every movement and release technique in this book at backhealer.com.

Use code AMAZON30 for 30% discount.

Suggested Reading

"Light on Pranyama" B.K.S. Iyengar

The definitive guide to yogic breathing from B.K.S. Iyengar, the world's most respected yoga teacher.B.K.S. Iyengar has devoted his life to the practice and study of yoga.

"Anatomy Trains" Thomas Myers , Melanie Burns, Cristy Harper

This book is a study guide for our foundational Anatomy Trains in Structure and Function course, and it eases the way with core concepts. Assimilation of BodyReading and application in movement and manual therapy is the work of a career.

Made in the USA
Monee, IL
04 November 2026

67391353R00075